'Russell has created a wonderfi
time truly recognised what coι
ituality on the stressful journε
Russell does not shy away fror   ......g ιпc significant stain
the fertility journey can have on a couples relationship. He offers
helpful and practical advice that can help a couple get through
the tough times and emerge with a stronger relationship whether
its with the child they so much desire or to build a meaningful ,
loving childless relationship with each other. This book is a must
read for all couples struggling with their fertility'

> **Dr Trevor Wing**, Medical Director of The Women's
> Natural Health Clinic, researcher and lecturer in
> gynaecological and obstetric healthcare for women.

This book is as valuable on you fertility journey as any good
road map or GPS when you are driving.

> **Michael Dooley,** Medical Director of the Poundbury
> Clinic, NHS Consultant Gynaecologist and a Fellow of
> the Royal College of Obstetricians and Gynaecologists.

'Russell is one of the most inspiring speakers I've encoun-
tered in the world of fertility and infertility. Now he's poured his
wisdom into a brilliant book. I love the easy to read chapters, the
sharing of his own story, along with his amazing advice and the
finest teachings of others. I know it will help so many people on
the roller-coaster of infertility - in fact more than that, on the
roller-coaster of life!'

> **Jessica Hepburn,** Author of The Pursuit of Motherhood
> and 21 Miles: swimming in search of the meaning of
> motherhood

'Russell has managed to cover the complicated rollercoaster that infertility presents in a gentle yet brilliantly informative and practical guide. I know from the many people I've spoken to about the stresses they endure whilst dealing with infertility that this book will be such a help. I'll definitely be shouting about it.'

Natalie Silverman, Host of The Fertility Podcast

Conceivable

'Get off the infertility emotional rollercoaster and fast-track your journey to getting pregnant whether naturally or with IVF.

Russell Davis

The information in this book is not intended as medical advice
or to replace a one-on-one relationship with a qualified health
care professional. It is intended as a sharing of knowledge and
information from the research and experience of Russell Davis.
We encourage you to make your own health care decisions based
upon your research and in partnership with a qualified health care
professional.

The author expressly disclaims any responsibility for any liability,
loss or risk, personal or otherwise, which is incurred as a result of
using any of the techniques or recommendations suggested here-
in. If in any doubt, or if requiring medical advice, please contact
the appropriate health care professional.

First edition

ISBN 978-1-5272-3847-3

To Bevan & Ewan

Contents

Foreword

After over 30 years of clinical care and research in the area of human fertility, I firmly believe that the management of your fertility is more than just pure clinical medicine.

The management of any issue in medicine requires medical input but also there are other essential areas that need to be addressed including ethical, emotional, financial, legal, friends, family and belief.

I wish CONCEIVABLE was around 30 years ago because it is a fantastic resource for both those trying to conceive and those caring for them. I wish I had read it 30 years ago.

I have known Russell for over 10 years and his book clearly demonstrates his professionalism and skill as a coach and Cognitive Hypnotherapist. It is well written and clear and very informative and to me, essential reading.

It addresses all the important areas of the mind

As Russell states life is a rollercoaster – so is the fertility journey. It needs careful planning clarity and understanding that they will be positive but also negative moments throughout the journey. In my opinion, the skill is to keep going and Russell could become your guardian angel on the journey. This book is as valuable on you fertility journey as any good road map or GPS when you are driving.

Thank you, Russell. I know my patients and my colleagues will benefit from your knowledge, experience wisdom and care.

Michael Dooley, Medical Director of the Poundbury Clinic, NHS Consultant Gynaecologist and a Fellow of the Royal College of Obstetricians and Gynaecologists.

Introduction

It's not uncommon to hear about couples that give up trying to conceive and then get pregnant out of the blue. We can imagine why that would be. We can imagine that our bodies relax and nature can take it's course more naturally when we are not stressed about whether another month is going to pass without success or whether this treatment is going to work or not.

It's well good knowing that it's better to be more relaxed but is that really possible? We can't trick ourselves in to not caring or 'giving up'.

Whether you are trying naturally or with fertility treatment I want to share what we learned on our 10-year fertility journey (and beyond) that if we knew at the beginning would have meant it would not have been a 10-year journey.

I've helped hundreds of women and couples to fast-track their journey to success and often to get pregnant against all odds.

My purpose of this book is to guide you to a place of peace, without giving up. Yes, it does exist. And actually, it's within you already. But I mustn't get ahead of myself.

The book is designed with small bite-sized chapters you can read and digest and dip back in to as a friend, encourager and guide on your journey.

With love

Russellx

Part 1

What keeps you on the rollercoaster

1

❖

How to read this book

As I sat in my seat in the second row (the front row felt too exposed) the music started and the speaker came up to the front of the room. I was looking forward to this workshop. I had spent a lot of money and effort to be there. I had my notebook and pen at the ready to capture the pearls of wisdom that I believed were going to make a difference in my own life as well as my work with my clients.

The speaker suggested we put our pads and pens down and have an 'experience' for the two days. My heart raced at even the idea of that. What if I would miss 'the' thing that made the difference! Surely I would forget the thought provoking quotes! How would I make sure I got the value I wanted from this time? However, I trusted the speaker and went along with it.

As I put my pad and pen down I felt naked. Something inside of me was telling me I wasn't taking the workshop 'seriously enough' by not making notes. I was thinking, how can I be concentrating fully on the content if I am not making notes to remember it all?

However, I had one of most profound experiences I've had at a training event. And because of this experience I've had many since.

I want to encourage you to do the same. I want to encourage you to read this book for an experience, not making notes, underlining or folding pages down. I want you to be aware of your internal feelings and insights as you read. Don't read for intellectual understanding, to reinforce what you think you know or to find out something you don't know, to find that magic bullet that is going to make everything OK for you.

When it comes to matters of the heart, intellectual thinking is not going to help you. It is a change of heart about where your well-being comes from and what is creating your experience moment to moment that will make the difference. Insights change lives.

How many times do we go to training, workshops or events and make loads of notes that make no difference to our lives (professionally or personally). It is better to have one 'aha' moment, one insight that makes a difference, than loads of written notes that you never refer back to.

You cannot force an insight. You cannot think your way to light-bulb moments. In fact as you will discover, it is your thinking that is causing your problem. You cannot fight thought with thought and it's not about changing negative thinking for more positive thinking. That rarely works and doesn't change lives.

We work so hard to succeed in life. You can probably look back at things you have achieved in your life and see how you worked hard and achieved your goal. However, that doesn't apply to having children, which can lead to frustration, despair and grief. You need a different approach, to your fertility journey, to life.

That starts with a different approach to this book. Stop trying so hard. Have an experience reading it, you can read it time and time again if you want. Don't try and 'get' it', read whilst being aware of a feeling within.

When you get an insight it is tempting to race on excitedly looking for another one. Slow things down. Sit with the insight, stop reading. For an insight to be life-changing you need to give it space to germinate and filtrate through your mind and soul. You get a change of heart about yourself and life. That's when an insight, a moment of understanding, can change your life.

I am about changing lives. Helping clients have a very different (and more peaceful) outlook and experience in all areas of their life. This enables them to have peace of mind wherever they are on their fertility journey. It enables their mind and body to relax, to come back to the present moment and be more aware of and tune in to their body and instinct. We bring our limiting thoughts and beliefs about ourselves to our fertility journey. For me, taking a step back from Project Baby and diving in to Project You for a short while means Project Baby takes more care of itself (with or without treatment). You can actually gain time doing this as you and your body fall in to the most healthy psychological and physical states.

For me, doing this not only accelerated our fertility journey (had we known then what we know now it would not have been a 10 year journey) as well as me being so much more content in who I am. I am sure I am a better father having had this learning and experience I am going to share with you in this book.

Let me be your guide on a journey. A journey to a place of peace without giving up. To KNOWING you are OK whatever happens. For life to begin to flow again even ahead of getting pregnant. It does exist. We found it on our journey.

That is where the magic can happen.

2

You're not alone

After being disillusioned by the traditional western approach to her PCOS of 'you just have to live with it and manage it with medication', my wife sought a more natural and holistic approach to her health and fertility. Over an eight-year journey including a change in lifestyle (letting go of stress), nutrition and holistic medicine, she, for the first time in her life, had a regular and healthy cycle. Having our own children was a now possibility. There was no reason to believe it wouldn't happen.

Up until that point, we had been telling ourselves we were OK with not having children. We are involved in youth and children's work, had a lot of godchildren, children were an important part of our lives in various ways. We always knew fostering or adoption may be an option and were open to that.

However, it wasn't until it became a real possibility that we were honest with ourselves about our desire to have our own children. Until then we had been kidding ourselves to protect us from the pain and disappointment. We began to accept the reality of our incredibly strong desire to be parents. The brave faces came off and we were in the front car of the fertility emotional roller-coaster.

After a year or so of trying with no success (as you know you become experts in human reproduction so know what you are doing!), for the first time it was suggested that I had a test. When I went to get the test results you can imagine my face when I was asked whether I had ever been exposed to dangerous levels of radiation. The results were that bad. Talk about a shock. Talk about a kick in the teeth. We thought we had run the marathon of infertility and were about to cross the finish line. It felt like we were now being told we would have to keep running and run another marathon, but an even tougher one. We were shell-shocked. Nothing had prepared us for this.

We started all the usual things to try and improve my fertility such as acupuncture, herbs, lifestyle, keeping my mobile phone out of my pocket, etc. However, deep down I think we knew it was pretty futile. It was going to need a miracle to raise my results off the floor to any reasonable level (count, morphology, and mobility!).

Bevan started going through the grieving process because in reality that is what we were doing, grieving the possibility of having our own children. Bevan was, I wasn't. I wasn't really acknowledging or accepting the reality of the situation. My grief, pain, and disillusionment.

My unwillingness to accept the reality of my infertility was trapping me in it. My wife was clearly on a journey to a place of acceptance and peace. She was moving to a place where she could continue the journey whilst feeling stronger, to a place where she could begin to imagine being fulfilled in the future, with or without children. It didn't mean she wanted children any less – she was born to parent, whether our own or others – it meant she could still imagine a fulfilling life without our own children. This would allow her to move on to the next phase of our journey (ICSI) in a much better place. I, however, felt I was stuck in avoidance and fear. Fearful of my own emotions.

I believe society doesn't really understand or accept the huge emotional impact struggling to have children can bring. It can lead to those experiencing infertility thinking they are wrong for feeling how they do.

There is nothing wrong with feeling how you do. It is natural. However, there is plenty we can do with those feelings to enable you to find peace of mind, without giving up the journey. Yes, that place does exist. It is also from this place you are more likely to get pregnant.

The lowest point of our fertility journey was the beginning of a personal journey that led me to that place of peace. That led me to review all aspects of my life and how I was living it. That led to us getting pregnant naturally against all odds (one in a billion, we were told, for it to happen naturally). It also lead me to be more of the man, husband, and father I want to be. They say out of our greatest pain can come our greatest gift. That is my wish for you through this book.

If we had known then what we know now it would not have been a 10 year journey.

And it's not just our story. I see it regularly with my clients. Chloe was diagnosed with polycystic ovaries, endometriosis, protein S deficiency and hormone imbalances. She had never ovulated regularly and has had problematic periods since puberty. Everything was stacked against her. After a failed IUI and IVF she was feeling very depressed, angry and bitter, spending a lot of time hiding in bed and crying. Her depression was getting worse as each month went by. She reached out from under the duvet. By helping her access her fertile mind she found a greater sense of peace within herself, more energy for life and went on to have twins with her next cycle of IVF.

It can be a lonely journey. Let me be your companion alongside you.

3

❖

'Project You' v 'Project Baby'

Through working with my clients and my own personal experience it has become clear to me that the thoughts, feelings and beliefs we experience on our fertility journey are not caused by or specific to our struggles in having our own children.. They are thoughts and beliefs we have about ourselves and life generally that we bring to our fertility journey.

If a client talks about their fear of not getting pregnant, when we explore that fear the intent behind it can be something like fear of failing. When we track this fear back into the past it has usually been in their life relating to other things, e.g. fear of failing to meet other expectations. So the fear has been there a lot of their life but the current thing it is being applied to is getting pregnant. Clients are often very surprised when we uncover these links. However, at the same time, they can see how it all makes sense.

When we start to recognise and uncover these background thoughts, feelings, and beliefs then we can begin to see a bigger shift in our fertility journey experience. Then we can really get off the emotional roller-coaster.

On our fertility journey, at our lowest point, I took myself to a convent to get away from life and 'be' in the pain and difficulties of infertility. I realised I had a tendency to avoid emotions. It was time to stop running.

As I sat in the beautiful convent gardens my gaze moved to two vegetable patches. One full of succulent vegetables – row upon row of lush green vegetation. The other – a scrubby patch of soil – a few lonely weeds the only sign of life.

Struck by the stark contrast between the two, my eyes came to rest upon the empty one. It felt like my life – barren and empty. Everyone else's life seemed to mirror the other one – vibrant and full of things that bring them happiness. Life appeared to be easier for them. For some reason, true happiness and contentment felt harder for me to achieve. "Perhaps I don't deserve life to be easy, or perhaps I haven't worked hard enough for the happiness they appear to access effortlessly." I thought.

I was not truly happy. This was a revelation for me. I had many pleasurable things in my life. I worked really hard – striving for the things in life that I believed bring happiness. The school grades. The degree. The successful career with the good pension. A lovely wife. Plenty of friends. A spiritual faith.

"How come I have so studiously done all my homework, been the good boy, and yet life seems like a continual struggle just to keep from feeling like something is missing?"

With a dying baby rabbit in my hand (I shall explain all later!) I made a decision: I am going on a journey. I am going to start living the life I want rather than the life I think others expect of me. I am going to do more things I enjoy just for the hell of it, to play more. 'Follow your bliss' is my mantra from now on!

I looked up at the vegetable patches. I looked at the empty one.

Yes, that is my life. It's not full of thriving vegetables, but it is a blank canvas: A fertile soil ready to support a new life for me.

We are so focussed on Project Baby when what would help us most is taking a step back and focussing on Project You. Seeing through the illusion of our habitual thoughts grants us a new perspective on circumstances. It gives us clarity. It gives us the inner strength we were born with. It frees us to re-connect to our innate well-being. These thoughts and beliefs are not who we are, habitual thought patterns about life and ourselves we have picked up along the way, particularly from childhood.

Some people are scared about moving their focus away from their fertility, taking their foot off the gas on Project Baby. Often this fear is because they're scared of their biological clock ticking. In my experience, taking a short time to focus on you, to find that place of peace without giving up, can buy you time. Being in the optimum state psychologically can help you be in the optimum state physically. There is a growing body of studies that are demonstrating the power of the mind and the body. The mind and body are one system. My wife and I got pregnant naturally against all odds; I've seen the same with my clients. Letting go of the undercurrent of fear, not deserving, or other limiting beliefs lets us flow again in life.

I tried everything to improve my fertility and nothing worked. Having had this experience and finding peace without giving up, within four months my wife was pregnant naturally against all odds whilst waiting to start an ICSI cycle. We weren't even trying because we were told there was no point. I did another test. My fertility had improved dramatically without me trying to improve it. My Project You journey had led me to being in a state of flow, and my body followed suit.

The more we focus on Project You, Project Baby takes more care of itself whether naturally or with treatment. This is my wish for your own journey, for your life, because Project You is not just about fertility, it is about you knowing you are OK in all of life. I believe I am a better father as a result of my own Project

You journey. I am far more content, have changed career and although I wouldn't wish a 10 year fertility journey on anyone, I am so thankful for what I learned about myself.

Project You can lead you to:

Relaxing into the journey KNOWING whatever happens you will be OK.

KNOWING you are truly loved and awesome for who you are; you have nothing to prove to anyone.

Not being scared of failing at anything in life.

Life beginning to flow again.

Your body falling in to the most healthy state for you to get pregnant!

Welcome to the beginning of your Project You!

4

Accepting it's tough

On our fertility journey, I often found it difficult to allow myself to feel the pain and sadness of childlessness. Part of me kept thinking that we have our health, a roof over our head, a good job, etc. and there are plenty of people in the world that don't have enough food to eat. How could I be down about not having children when we are warm, safe and secure?

Then there are well-meaning friends and family trying to be supportive, saying things like 'just relax and things will be OK'. They just didn't understand and I didn't feel able to open up and express how I really felt.

I also thought I had to stay strong and hopeful otherwise it would never happen. I believed losing hope and falling apart would mean defeat and I was not ready for that. I couldn't imagine a happy life without children. I was striving for the finish line, trying to stay strong and positive but in doing so part of me wasn't accepting how tough the journey was. I thought that was a sign of weakness and would mean I would give up, collapse under the strain and distress.

However, it's really tough, isn't it? It can be harder to accept that when no-one around you understands what you are experiencing. Most people can never understand the depth of stress and distress this journey can bring unless they have experienced it. A 1993 study[1] by Harvard Medical School revealed just how distressing infertility can be. The study showed that the levels of anxiety and depression in women with infertility were only slightly lower than those of women with AIDS and chronic pain. It equalled those of women with conditions such as cancer, hypertension and heart disease. And no-one tells them just to relax!

Another study[2] showed 63% of women who had experienced both rated infertility as being more stressful than divorce.

So you are not weak for feeling sad, angry or defeated.

Accepting the reality of a situation is key to creating something new. A marathon runner can accept the pain but it doesn't mean they are giving up.

Accepting reality is part of the creation process. You cannot create anything without first accepting where you are now. When we try and ignore the pain and pretend things are different, perhaps with positive affirmations, we are often kidding ourselves.

If you wake up feeling emotionally empty and try and lift yourself by telling yourself 'you're ok' you are more likely trying to trick yourself, resisting the reality of the situation. This is neither helpful nor realistic. It is underpinned by a belief that you are a failure or wrong for feeling that way and you should be feeling more positive in order to be successful.

During our fertility journey, I felt disillusioned about life. I felt angry and fearful about never being happy. I was in a job I didn't enjoy but it paid well and was convenient. I was not accepting the reality that I was not happy in life in general, including in my marriage. Life wasn't living up to the expectations I had of it. Keeping my head in the sand kept me from doing anything about it. It was familiar. I had worked in the same company all my working life and I was scared of changing; what happens if I move and the new job is worse? As I began exploring this, accepting my feelings, it enabled me to begin the process of creating something different and finding something I love doing.

It was the same with our fertility. I was not accepting the pain, anger and fear that was inside me. For a long time, I felt I had to be the 'strong one', ignoring my emotions to be there for my wife. As we shall explore in more detail later, this had the opposite effect. What she wanted was me to be honest and feel emotionally connected, that is what creates unity. Hiding my emotions was doing the opposite. Unbeknown to me, it was also impacting my fertility.

Allow whatever shows up to show up. What if you didn't need to be scared of any experience? My intent is by the end of this book you are not scared of any of your experiences – not just on your fertility journey, in life as a whole.

Acceptance is the WD40 of change. Once you allow what is to be you can begin to move on from it. You cannot leave a place you've never been to. Not that I believe you have to weep and wail to let an emotion go. However, resistance just makes it stronger.

What can stop us accepting and being is fear of running out of time. Fear of not having time to accept. One of my first fertility clients, Michelle, many years ago had just completed her third IVF cycle, which was unsuccessful. She sat in my clinic just completely exhausted. Worn out emotionally and physically. Although unsuccessful, many aspects of this cycle were very positive and the clinic recommended another round of IVF with a revised protocol.

Being 39, Michelle feared time was running out so felt she had to go straight in to the next round. She also felt unspoken pressure from her husband and family who believed that they were so close to being successful they needed to try again as soon as possible.

As we talked it dawned on her that it related to my analogy of the marathons. She had run three marathons only to get to the end of each one and be told she had to start again. She had just finished her third on the trot and she had nothing left physically and emotionally to give. It was OK for her supporters, they were standing alongside the route and cheering. She was the one that had to do the running. Her mind and body needed time to relax, recover and heal, despite the ticking clock in her head.

Her first bit of therapy was to tell her to have a 'fertility holiday'. To take some time off from her emotional marathon running. Having equipped her with some restorative hypnosis tracks, I told her to come back when she felt ready to. I am pleased to say she took that to heart. Returning two months later, she was looking and feeling so much stronger, ready for us to prepare her mind and body for her fourth IVF cycle the following month, which was successful. Taking a fertility holiday can buy you time biologically, not waste it. It can put your mind in to a much healthier psychological state, which puts your body in to a much healthier physical state. Michelle harvested a much higher number of good quality eggs in her 4th cycle compared to her previous ones. Was it purely down to a change in protocol? Michelle doesn't believe so. She said she felt so different psychologically she is convinced it made a difference biologically.

Allow yourself to accept how tough it is. Be kind to yourself in this moment. The more you honour yourself and your body the more you and your body can fall in to the healthiest state for you to get pregnant.

1. Domar AD, Zuttermeister PC, Friedman R. *Journal of Psychosomatic Obstetrics and Gynecology*. 1993; 14: 45–52.

2. Mahlstedt PP, MacDuff S, Bernstein J. *Emotional factors in the in vitro fertilisation and embryo transfer process. J. In Vitro Embryo Transfer*. 1987; 4: 323–6.

5

What is acceptance?

I came to the realisation I had a dustbin full of emotions I was avoiding with a heavy brick on the lid. The anger and sadness of our journey were touching on the same emotions of what I had (unconsciously) put in my bin from childhood. So naturally, I avoided the grief, sadness, and anger of childlessness.

My wife was processing her emotions, her grief, and it was clear I was not. I became aware I was not really feeling anything. I had glimpses of feelings but most of the time I was not in touch with them. I filled my life with distractions (such as work, internet, thinking) to avoid the feelings. You cannot think and feel at the same time and I spent a lot of time thinking. I had a very busy mind. This prevented me from feeling not just emotions, such as the pain and sadness, but even happiness and joy when good things happened in life. I flat-lined through life. For others who have a busy mind, it means they can flip from thinking into strong feelings. The over-thinking can fuel and sustain very strong emotions. What's behind the emotions is all the over-thinking.

I decided I couldn't go on like this, it wasn't helping me, my wife or our relationship. I realised I had to stop running from my feelings. I needed to take myself away from all my distractions and just be, and allow whatever needed to come up to come. I took myself to a convent for a week. Living in simplicity with the nuns away from the internet, work, and life. This was not something I had ever done before, however I instinctively knew it was what I needed. To strip away the distractions of life and be with myself for long enough to allow and accept whatever feelings arose.

So, one day as I sat in the convent's beautiful gardens contemplating the difficulties of life, one of the nuns approached me. Out of the blue, she handed me a small bundle of fur. It was a baby rabbit that had been caught by one of the nuns' many cats. She didn't know what to do about it, so brought it to me. At first, I was annoyed. "Why has she given it to me? I am here to get some space for reflection and to be left alone."

I looked down at the tiny rabbit cupped in my hands with its soft brown fur and its eyes looking up at me. It was panting rapidly. I could not see any obvious signs of injury but it was clearly in a state of distress. I was pretty sure it was going to die.

As I looked at this beautiful, helpless little creature, I felt an immense wave of sadness. I couldn't bear the thought of it dying alone. I know I was engaging in anthropomorphism, but I couldn't help the wave of sadness and grief building up inside of me. "Does this little baby rabbit know it is loved?" I didn't want it to die alone not knowing. I began to cry. The crying turned to sobbing. It surprised me because I usually live in my head so I don't have to feel my emotions. I sobbed for this rabbit, but of course, I was really sobbing for me. The lid had come off my bin.

"Do I feel loved?"

"Do I allow myself to be loved?"

I knew on a conscious level that my wife loved me, my family and friends, but how loved do I feel?

"Do I really KNOW it in my heart?"

The answer was a resounding "No!"

For the rest of my time at the convent I became more aware

of my feelings about all sorts of areas of my life. Being in a job that was not fulfilling, infertility, my past.

For the first time, I accepted my feelings, my unhappiness at work, my anger and the pain of infertility.

It was only in recognising and accepting the reality of the situation could I begin to move on. I came away from that time beginning to find a sense of peace about life and even infertility. That doesn't mean I had given up all hope or no longer wanted children, far from it, but I felt more peaceful about being able to have a fulfilled life whatever happened. I know that sounds impossible but believe me, it can be done. I felt ready to take the next step on our journey, to start exploring fertility treatment (ICSI) with a deep longing for children but also with a sense of peace and well-being about the future regardless of the outcome.

Accepting a situation is not resigning to believe things are never going to change. Accepting is not denying your own needs, wishes, and desires. Far from it. Acceptance is not giving up.

Acceptance is letting go of the stories you are telling yourself about the situation and future, e.g. 'It's never going to change'. Nothing can predict the future. Not even your thinking.

Acceptance is letting go of the thinking you have about yourself, e.g. 'I don't deserve...'

Acceptance is letting go of judgments, e.g. 'It's not fair' – they're just thoughts/stories you are choosing to believe.

Acceptance is accepting reality and finding self-compassion for yourself in that reality.

Accepting is seeing you are OK in this moment. It doesn't mean you don't want things to be different, it means at this moment, the only moment that exists, you are OK. You have food in the fridge, the love from friends and family, you are OK in this moment.

Lack of acceptance of ourselves and reality keeps us strapped in the emotional roller-coaster. It's this emotional roller-coaster that keeps tension and stress in our bodies which is not going to be helping your chances of getting pregnant.

Try this exercise. Put your hand on your heart and say out loud, 'I accept myself as I am today'. And then just notice what feelings or thoughts come to mind. Do you accept yourself fully? How would it feel if you did?

6

Hope v acceptance

What is hope?

Is it a good thing? Surely having hope is a good thing.

Hope helps you stay positive, doesn't it?

Hope keeps away despair and fear, doesn't it?

Hope can often be fuelled by fear. Fearful thinking that something won't (or will) happen.

Hope can go beyond wanting, towards longing and needing, underpinned by fear and perhaps even desperation.

Hope and fear are possibly two sides of the same coin.

Just like you can't have anger without love (you can't be angry with someone you don't care about). The opposite of love is not anger, it's indifference. The opposite of fear is not hope or belief, it's acceptance.

Acceptance doesn't mean giving up. You know you can continue your journey without fear or desperation because when we're in the here and now we recognise we have everything we need, in this moment.

Hope is future thinking. Any thinking that is not in the present moment is fantasy. The future does not exist except in our thinking.

I can remember all too well wishing and hoping things were different on our fertility journey. Longing for things to be different. I prayed and prayed to God/life/the universe (for me back then it was God) to be blessed with the gift of a child. For happiness I believe we so deserved. For a break from the heartache and struggle life had felt for so long.

That longing continued until I found peace and acceptance. A place of peace without giving up (it does exist, trust me!).

We could then continue our journey, still wanting to have a baby but without the fear of it not happening. Without the need for hope. Because you don't need hope when in the here and now. As humans we are built to be in and thrive in the here and now. We have everything we need in the here and now. We don't need hope in the present moment.

7

Stress and fertility

Conception is one of the most delicate systems in the human body. It requires a delicate cocktail of hormones that need to be in balance and continuously changing throughout the cycle. The delicate balance is vulnerable to stress, obesity, diet, exercise, and many other factors. Let's look at how our emotions, particularly stress in its many forms can impact your fertility.

Unfortunately, the fight-or-flight alarm reaction engages both the hypothalamus and the pituitary gland, both of which also function to regulate the proper balance of fertility hormones required for the reproductive system. It shuts down non-critical systems. It has to ensure everything is focussed on survival.

This survival mechanism is designed to enable us to overcome short term threats to our well-being. When the threat has passed or we have successfully escaped/fought it off the system settles back down to the status quo and all bodily functions quickly return to normal.

The problem arises when stress becomes more chronic and the fight-or-flight response remains activated long term. This causes an ongoing impact to the hypothalamus and pituitary gland (and consequently the production of FSH and LH). The increased level of adrenaline begins to disrupt the activity of progesterone, another key hormone for reproduction.

The raised level of cortisol during prolonged periods of stress has also been shown to inhibit implantation of a fertilised egg into the lining of the uterus. Prolactin levels also rise when the body is under stress which can prevent ovulation from even taking place.

While in this state of hyper-alertness for survival, blood is also being automatically diverted to the muscles in order to maximise the body's ability to either fight off or flee from the stressor. This is at the expense of other systems including both the digestive and reproductive systems impacting their functioning and over time this can actually lead to a thinning of the uterine wall lining.

On top of all this, at times of stress you may notice how you lose your sex drive; you are tired & stressed and it is probably the last thing on your mind. As you would expect if you're facing a sabre tooth tiger!!

One of the reasons for this is that when stress continues for too long it impacts the adrenal glands and you can get what is known as adrenal burn-out. They begin to lose their ability to secrete DHEA (dehydroepiandrosterone) which is an important hormone and is required for the production of oestrogen, progesterone and testosterone and is necessary for maintaining a balance of these sex hormones within the body. Consequently, a decrease in the level of DHEA not only leads to a decrease in sex drive in both genders, it can also become a major causative factor in both menstrual problems and infertility in women.

The medical world is split as to whether stress is a cause of infertility. In my experience, both personal and with clients, I (and they) firmly believe it is. This echoes a growing body of research that indicates stress can have a direct impact on natural conception fertility and IVF success.

In research[1] published in *Fertility and Sterility* in 2004, experts at the University of California at San Diego reported that stress may play a role in the success of infertility treatments, including in vitro fertilisation (IVF). After administering a series of questionnaires designed to measure patients' stress levels, the researchers found that women who scored highest (indicating the highest levels of stress) had ovulated 20% fewer eggs compared with women who were less stressed. Moreover, of those who were able to produce eggs, those who were most stressed were 20% less likely to achieve fertilisation success.

Another study[2] by researchers at Oxford University and the US National Institute of Health provides evidence for the first time of an association between high levels of stress and reduced chances of a woman conceiving during the fertile days of her monthly cycle. The study included data from 274 healthy women aged between 18 and 40 who were trying to become pregnant. During the study, the women provided saliva samples on day 6 of each of their menstrual cycles to test for levels of the hormone cortisol and alpha-amylase (an indicator of adrenalin/stress levels). The results showed that the chances of getting pregnant for the quarter of women in the study with the highest levels (top 25%) of alpha-amylase were roughly 12% lower than the quarter of women with the lowest levels of alpha-amylase, each day during the fertile days of their menstrual cycle. Interestingly, no differences in the chances of becoming pregnant were found for women with different levels of cortisol so it appears that adrenaline may be the stress hormone which affects fertility the most.

This can appear to be all doom and gloom. It's pretty impossible to avoid feeling stressed on this fertility journey. However, keep reading because it's not as bad as you think. Yes, stress can have a huge impact on your chances of getting pregnant, however, it doesn't need to be that way. And on the flip side, just think of the possibilities for you and your body if you could let go of any negative impact stress and distress may be having on your chances of getting pregnant?

Klonoff-Cohen H, Natarajan L. *Fertility and Sterility.* 2004; 81(4): 982-998

2. Buck Louis GM, Lum KJ, Sundaram R, Chen Z, Kim S, Lynch CD, Schisterman EF, Pyper C. *Fertility and Sterility.* 2011; 95 (7): 2184-2189

8

❖

Understanding stress

So stress is not good for your chances of getting pregnant let alone your experience of the journey. However, you probably knew that and want to know how to stop being stressed! We will get on to that. But first I want to look at stress a little more. Believe it or not stress itself is not a problem for us and our bodies. It's our stress about being stressed! The more we understand the true nature of stress and not being scared of the fact we may be feeling stress at any point in time, it will have little or no hold over us. It moves on so much quicker and doesn't have a negative impact on our bodies and chances of getting pregnant.

Stress is there to keep us safe. Safe from physical dangers. To keep us on high alert ready to respond to the threat. To attack or run away. To fight or flight. Hence being called the fight or flight response. It keeps you safe when walking down a dark alley at night. Keeps you vigilant to potential dangers. It keeps you safe if you are walking too close to a cliff edge on a coast path.

The stress response gets you ready for action. Gets your heart pumping faster to get the blood to our muscles ready for the fight or flight. It floods our body with stress hormones that give us the short burst of energy, power, and strength needed to deal with the threat.

When the human mind perceives that it is undergoing a stressful event it sets off an alarm reaction initiated by the hypothalamus. The hypothalamus immediately recruits both the pituitary gland at the base of the brain and the adrenal glands situated on top of the kidneys.

These glands immediately begin to flood the bloodstream with a cocktail of stress hormones including adrenaline to prepare the body for what is referred to as the 'fight-or-flight' response.

The 'fight-or-flight' response, or the Sympathetic Nervous System to give it its technical name, is just that, preparing the body to fight the danger or run from it. It goes back to the hunter-gatherer in us and is a response all mammals have. It is controlled by a primitive part of our brain, the mammalian part of our brain called the limbic system. Our brain has evolved over the years from the reptilian brain which controls the most basic life support systems. The brain then evolved and formed the mammalian or limbic system where behaviour is less rigidly controlled by instincts. Feelings such as attachment, anger, and fear emerge with associated behavioural response patterns of freeze, fight, or flight. The hypothalamus in the limbic system maintains the body's status quo, receiving inputs about blood pressure, body temperature, hunger, thirst, fluid and electrolyte balance, circadian rhythms and initiating any necessary changes to maintain proper balances.

The third element of the brain's development is the neo-cortex found in humans (and whales and dolphins!). It controls higher order thinking skills, reason and speech, and our various types of intelligence (music, math, spatial conceptualisation, intuition, imagination, etc.).

So the fight-or-flight response prepares us for action. It is controlled by the primitive area of our brain as it doesn't want to be slowed down by logical arguments or thought. If you see a large ferocious dog running towards you looking like it's going to attack, standing there thinking about who owns the dog, wondering where the owner is, whether it is really going to attack your or not or whether it has seen a cat behind you, isn't going to help you, is it? Your fight-or-flight response kicks in and immediately prepares you to get out of the way or do what you need to do to protect yourself. Its function is to protect us and maximise the body's ability to survive the stressful event. The stress hormones get the blood pumping around our body ready for activity, increases our breathing rate to ensure our muscles have enough oxygen for activity and we are on high-alert ready to respond.

Have you ever heard of the amazing stories of women being able to lift a car to save their child trapped underneath in the aftermath of an accident? This miraculous feat of strength is possible due to the cocktail of stress hormones giving extra power and strength in those times when most needed, times of survival.

We don't encounter sabre-tooth tigers or car accidents day to day, however our brain responds in the same way to psychological stress – it cannot differentiate between the two, for the mammalian brain stress is stress.

What is perceived as stressful will vary from person to person. We all find different things stressful. For me following a recipe can be stressful! For others, it's a walk in the park.

In our modern, fast-paced lives, the amount of background stress people have is on the increase. We may not be consciously aware of what we are feeling stressed about or it may be something that tips it over the edge and we find our response to a situation feels stronger than it warrants. It's because the emotion coming out is not really about the current situation.

I remember a video going around on the internet of a woman going berserk at a McDonald's drive-through window because they didn't have any chicken McNuggets. Of course, it wasn't about the chicken McNuggets, it was the straw that broke the camel's back. The stress response stays on for one situation and then with each additional stress not only does it pump the stress hormones around our body, it increases the expectation that stress is going to occur, becoming hyper-sensitive to it. We develop a fear of the fear. We become anxious about being anxious.

We have already looked at how fertility can be a huge source of stress, probably the biggest in your life.

The stress response works like a car alarm designed to keep us safe by warning of danger in our immediate environment. You could wonder why we have it if we are no longer threatened by sabre tooth tigers whilst hunting and gathering. But if you think about it, it is dangerous to turn it off completely, it would be like walking through the backstreets of a dark city at night without any fear signal.

However, just like a car alarm, it could also be oversensitive, people stop paying attention to it and it becomes very annoying. But being in a constant state of alert not only is exhausting, it can have some pretty serious health consequences, such as impacting your immune system in addition to affecting the delicate cocktail of hormones required for successful pregnancy. The pituitary gland in the brain controls the levels of stress hormones and fertility hormones.

It is possible to reset the sensitivity, to turn it down to a more appropriate and healthy level.

Just by understanding what stress is and how it works can be helpful in re-calibrating the stress response. It may help you to begin to re-interpret your thinking about the situation (the 'threat'). A situation in itself does not make you stressed; nothing can make you feel anything. It is you thinking about it, your perception of it that creates your internal experience. We shall explore this more later.

Learning stress reduction techniques can help you let go of stress in any given moment and turn off the stress response and allow the hormone and chemical balance in your system to return to a normal and healthy state, letting the adrenalin levels subside.

The body indicates it cannot take anymore, perhaps through headaches, being irritable, not sleeping well or seeking relief, maybe through food, alcohol or drugs.

The good news is when we understand more about the true nature of emotions such as stress and are no longer anxious about being stressed, the stress itself cannot hurt us. In fact, stress can be a catalyst for growth, helping us be more of the person we want to be. A lobster grows too big for its shell. It undergoes a period of being compressed, its body under stress. It feels uncomfortable. It goes off and finds somewhere to hide, perhaps under a rock, and sheds the shell and grows a new one. Until the next time. I don't suppose it panics about feeling that sensation of compression and stress. It sees it as a signal for growth. It has a different relationship with it.

The journey I want to take you on is to help you understand the true nature of stress and not be scared of it. Research on stress shows it only has an impact on us physically if we think it does, i.e. if we are stressed about being stressed. How would your fertility journey be different if you didn't have to be scared of any experience you were having, including stress?

Whether it's stress or whatever emotion we are experiencing, the more we understand what's creating it (our perception of life at that moment, not reality) the less of a hold it has over us and it moves on more quickly than you imagine.

9

❖

Allowance

So, if acceptance is the WD40 of change, what do I really mean by acceptance? What do we actually mean by any word we use? We all have our own deeper understanding and experience of a word. Acceptance can for some mean there is something 'bad' or 'negative' in their life they have to accept. That it's got to be endured. In my mind that's not fully accepting it. Another word that may convey what I mean by acceptance is allowance. Allowing whatever is without any judgement, resistance or resentment.

As adults, we are often trying to manage our state, how we feel. We don't enjoy feeling what we label as negative feelings such as sadness, fear, and anger. We want to have more 'positive' feelings such as happiness and peace. We are addicted to feeling comfortable. That's because part of us thinks we are not OK unless we feel OK. We think our feelings are telling us something is wrong.

We want to know what's making us feel bad so we know what we need to do to stop feeling that way. This response to feelings leads us to spend more and more time in the low mood. Trying harder and harder to be OK. We think we are trying to help ourselves be better but we are actually digging a bigger hole.

We tend to think our feelings are telling us something about us or our circumstances. We tend to say 'I am feeling X because of...' We look for the cause and if we cannot find it we get caught in our head looking for it. This is a misunderstanding of what a feeling is and what creates it.

A feeling is an expression of thought in our bodies. That's it. A feeling doesn't know anything about our circumstances or us (our capabilities, past etc.). Nothing makes us feel anything. We are not feeling our circumstances or who we are. We are feeling our thinking about that. 100% of our experience comes from thought.

We grow up thinking feelings are like a barometer. They are there to tell us something about us or life. Like a warning system. This is a misunderstanding of the nature of a feeling. Feelings don't know anything about our circumstances. They are thought being expressed in consciousness. Thoughts and feelings are two sides of the same coin.

Our emotions are like the speedometer of a car. The speedo has one job. It knows how fast the car is going. That's it. It doesn't know how hard the engine is working or how hot the engine is. It has one job and one job only. It's the same with our feelings; they know one thing. How much thinking we've got in this moment. That's it. They don't know what our circumstances are and they cannot feel the past or future as it doesn't exist.

If it were circumstances creating our experience then our experience would be constant until the circumstances changed. But it doesn't work like that. Some days are better than others. If it were the circumstances that create our experience everyone would have the same experience of a situation. Again it doesn't work like that; everyone has their own experience of it.

The more we understand the true nature of emotions the less we care about our feelings. The more we can allow them knowing they mean nothing about us or life. It means we have some sad, angry or fearful thinking at that moment. And left to their own devices thoughts come and go.

There is no solution to a feeling. It doesn't need a solution or changing in any way. Left to its own devices it'll move on.

So it's not the feeling that's the problem. We can't control our thinking, thus we cannot control what emotions we have. It's our relationship to our feelings that causes is the problem. It's whether we think it matters. As soon as we resent it, try and change it or even wish we weren't having it we are adding more thought into the mix, we are putting more energy into it. We get trapped on the rollercoaster. Left to its own devices thought always moves on and fresh perspectives come in. We move back to peace and clarity. It's how we are designed.

A minor example of this was I was out running on a cold winters morning. The wind was blowing ice cold rain on my face. My immediate response was to hunch up. My head went down and my shoulders went up. This can be how I respond energetically when I am not allowing my experience in the moment. When I collapse and go into my head resenting and fighting reality. I caught myself doing this on this run. So I allowed myself to fully feel the weather. I put my shoulders down and head up. I embraced it. Before I knew it I had forgotten all about it. My mind had gone on to something else. By the time my attention came back to the weather I was noticing how much it had changed, the rain had stopped and blue sky was breaking through the clouds.

It's the same with any human experience, any emotion. What you resist persists. What if there is no need to resist? It moves on like a weather system. You couldn't hold on to any experience forever even if you wanted to.

How would you be on this journey if you could fully allow any experience you are having, knowing it knows nothing about you, your circumstances or your future?

10

Anger

I was very angry with God/life/the universe/mother nature (whatever words work for you) on our fertility journey. To me, it just wasn't fair. Everyone else seemed to get what they wanted with much more ease. Life seemed so much harder for me, and it wasn't fair.

I've been more aware recently how I still have anger in me from childhood experiences. It's more of an undercurrent of resentment and frustration rather than rage. I had a lot of resentment towards my mother for the way she was when we were growing up. I have let much of that go which transformed my relationship with her for which I am ever grateful. However, I've been aware that I am still carrying some and it isn't serving me.

This anger that I have been holding, although is all related to past stuff, it contaminates my present experience. It is too easy for me to project this anger onto my wife by being in a bad mood or bring it into situations where it's not relevant (but sure looks like it is at the time!).

Anger dis-empowers us. It makes us feel like a victim because we are angry at the entity, person or situation that we think has made us angry. That has power over our state of being in some way. This can leave you feeling stuck in the feeling of anger and powerless to feel any different.

Anger also disconnects us. It stops us feeling connected to

our loved ones, to life and the present moment. It stops us from having peace and happiness.

Though I don't believe we have to weep and wail to let an emotion go. At the end of the day, emotions are thoughts, stories tell we are ourselves in this moment. But the more we understand what is creating our experience of anger – that it's not us or our situation but thoughts in this moment – we don't have to be scared of it. I judged myself as being bad for feeling angry. I thought it was destructive when actually suppressing it is more destructive as I end up being passive-aggressive.

It is our relationship with our emotions that cause more harm than the emotion itself. The emotion itself is neutral. It's a thought in this moment. It's when we judge ourselves for having it, or resent it or even resist it that it can have more power and become more destructive.

I've been using a Kundalini yoga practice to allow my anger and not be scared of it. It's like punching a pillow without the punching! Afterwards, I feel so open and receptive to the world. So much more available to give and receive love. To see the universe as a loving and supportive energy behind life.

What's your relationship with anger or other emotions? To resist them? Do you resent yourself for having them? Can you see it's your reaction to them that takes you on a journey further away from peace keeping you on the emotional roller-coaster?

11

Life is...

Finish this statement. Life is a...

We bring our thinking about ourselves and life to our fertility journey, we don't create new beliefs about ourselves and life within it. Although it can feel that way. It can be such an emotional journey it can shine a spotlight on the thoughts and beliefs about ourselves and life we had already. In the midst of our journey, I became aware of my belief that I wasn't truly loved for who I was. My clients find similar thoughts and beliefs come to the surface in our work together.

One of the things I am most grateful for about our fertility journey is that I learnt so much about myself and how I saw and engaged with life. Being aware of where my experiences were coming from (my limiting thoughts and beliefs) has enabled me to change all areas of my life for the better. It doesn't mean life's a breeze, but it means I am able to be more me, being more true to my soul rather than the people pleaser I was. Desperate for people to like me. Being more self-aware makes life a journey of growth and development rather than being stuck as a prisoner of my beliefs, thinking that was me & life and it cannot change.

You may have seen the bumper sticker, 'Life's a bitch and then you die'. This is a classic example of the powerless, victim (prisoner) of life mentality. Let's explore this philosophy a little more.

If we were to agree with the first statement, life is a bitch or any variation of it, such as life is a struggle or life is unfair, then why is dying and getting out of the prison of struggle such a bad thing? Surely it should be 'Life's a bitch but then you die!' with a positive inflection at the end! Otherwise it is a contradiction and creates what is called a double bind. It binds you into a circular argument that you cannot escape from.

Many people live life by this philosophy, without being consciously aware of it. I used to. I spent many years in a job that didn't inspire me whilst at the same time was scared I might be laid off when we went through rounds of redundancy. Many people feel the same about their life, their jobs or their relationships. When I finally took the step to leave out of choice to find a job that's more 'me' I lost count of the people that said to me they wished they could do the same. What was different about me from them? I had no super-powers or shed-loads of money to fall back on! It was their victim mentality that kept them trapped there.

In a poll of middle managers the most common response to the request to complete the statement 'Life's a...' was 'Life's a battle'. The most common response for business owners and executives was 'Life's a game'.

Things happen in life that we don't have control over. Life is a contact sport but we can see that as being a battle or a game. It becomes a battle if we think our survival or even psychological well-being is dependant on it. Dependent on outcomes we have no control over.

When things happen to us, without us having any choice, we do have a choice as to how we respond to it. The victim thinks they are powerless. The creator asks themselves 'what could I create from this situation?'

When we get stuck in traffic I can easily be frustrated and annoyed, telling myself there is nothing we can do, we are missing out on what we could be doing if we weren't stuck in this traffic.

Talk about being a victim. So now I ask myself, what do I want to create from this situation? If I am with the family it can be a time of playing some games or making up stories. If I am on my own it could be a time to listen to an audiobook or dictate some more of this book!

You may be thinking that's OK if what we are now going to be late for is not 'important'. This goes back to where we think our 'OKness' comes from, which we'll explore more later. What if you knew you were OK, no less of a human being, equal to others whether you are late for a meeting or not? What if your sense of OKness wasn't dependant on what others thought or external circumstances?

The turning point of our fertility journey was when we realised we could create a happy and meaningful life with or without children. Our preference was absolutely with, but it doesn't mean it cannot be done without. When we believe our well-being and happiness is dependent on external circumstances that is when we get caught in feeling, such as anxiety, depression or hopelessness, because we are looking in the wrong place and in a place where we have no control.

So we created our plan. To pack up and go travelling, with the dog, in a camper van. Have an adventure. We chose to use the freedom and flexibility our situation had provided to create something, an adventure. As it turned out we didn't get to go on the big adventure as we became pregnant naturally before we went – but not before the shift in mindset from victim to creator.

Creating a baby is the ultimate act of creating. How can you start creating in life today, even from within your current situation? What could you create that feels inspiring, whether something big or small doesn't matter, from your situation as it stands today?

12

Emotional needs audit

The Human Givens approach to therapy is based on a list of 'givens' or emotional needs of humans. The theory is if any of these needs are not met then it could impact our emotional well-being and can lead to stress, anxiety and disharmony in life.

When you look at these needs I think it highlights why infertility can be so stressful, lonely and such an emotionally exhausting journey.

The emotional needs audit rates how well your emotional needs are being met in your life right now, on a scale of one to seven (where one means not met at all and seven means being very well met):

- Do you feel secure in all major areas of your life? For instance, in your home life, work life or environment?
- Do you feel you receive enough attention?
- Do you think you give other people enough attention?
- Do you feel in control of your life most of the time?
- Do you feel part of the wider community?
- Can you obtain privacy when you need to?
- Do you have at least one close friend?
- Do you have an intimate relationship in your life? (i.e. you are totally accepted physically and emotionally for who you are by at least one person?)

- Do you feel an emotional connection to others?
- Do you have a status in life (whatever it may be) that you value and that is acknowledged?
- Are you achieving things in your life that you are proud of?
- Do you feel competent in at least one major area of your life?
- Are you mentally and/or physically stretched in ways which give you a sense of meaning and purpose?

If you scored any need three or less it is likely to be a major cause of stress in your life. If your experience is anything like my experience of infertility you may have scored pretty low in a number of them! I know I can look back on our fertility journey and see how these needs were not being met in me.

Let's take a look at each one in turn from the perspective of infertility.

Do you feel secure in all major areas of your life? For instance, in your home life, work life or environment?

"No." It can be hard to feel secure when the things you want and plan for do not happen and you feel you have very little control over it. The stress of infertility can impact all areas of your life whether relationships or work which again can affect the sense of security. Will my partner stay with me if we cannot have children? All sorts of doubts and insecurities can creep in.

Do you feel you receive enough attention?

"Yes, of the wrong type." You are probably lacking in emotional affection, are fed up with the humiliating attention from clinicians and do not get enough supportive attention from friends (because they just don't understand).

Do you think you give other people enough attention?

"I have nothing else to give, I am physically and emotionally drained." I often liken infertility to being like a marathon but every time you get another BFN it is like being told at the finish line you have to go back to the start and do it all again.

Do you feel in control of your life most of the time?

"No". It is very common to feel you have no control of your fertility; you are trying everything but nothing seems to be working. Your life is effectively on hold, you may even have stopped working to reduce some of the stress in your life so you no longer feel in control of your career. You may be worried about the cost of treatment, which again means you feel less in control of your finances.

Do you feel part of the wider community?

"No, I feel very isolated." It is surprising how isolating infertility can be. It is something that is so personal and misunderstood by friends/family it can be difficult to find people you can connect with honestly and be real with. There are plenty of online communities which is great, however, they are no substitute for real connections in your community. In so many ways local communities are centred around having children whether the ante-natal group continuing to meet, young mums meeting for coffee, the community at the school gate etc. You may be seeing friends building new communities since having children which means you could feel left out.

Can you obtain privacy when you need to?

"At times." Whether you have children or not is quite a public thing. There is an unspoken expectation from friends and family that you will have children and when you don't it is quite hard to hide the fact you haven't! 'So are you planning to have children' becomes a more common question than you think when you hit your mid 30s, as if the message behind the comment is 'you'd better get on with it before it's too late'. If someone asked us outright like that we were honest saying 'we don't think we can have children' being quite vague about the details and absolutely not saying whether it was a problem with myself or my wife (in the end it ended up being one then the other!). Now there's a conversation killer for you!

Do you have at least one close friend?

"Yes but even they don't really understand." Most of our closest friends just didn't understand what it was like not to be able to have children. I guess it is not until you cannot have something you truly understand how much you want it, and until you have been in the position of not being able to have it you cannot appreciate what it is like. We were lucky to also have some close friends who really took the time to listen and understand what it was like and we are also indebted to have friends who were on a similar journey – however, I am aware of how lucky we were to have this support. I encourage you to find someone you can really be honest with, someone who will take the time to listen and understand without judgement or assumptions.

Do you have an intimate relationship in your life? (i.e. you are totally accepted physically and emotionally for who you are by at least one person?)

"Yes, but we seem to have lost some of the intimacy recently." I believe one of the most unspoken aspects of infertility is the impact on your relationship with your partner/spouse. The strain on both of you is huge and this can inevitably affect your relationship if you do not take steps to ensure it doesn't. At a time when you want to feel closest to your partner, to be united in the journey, you may be feeling frustrated and disappointed that it isn't that way. I can speak from a male perspective – I thought the best thing for me was to be the 'strong one', that one of us had to be. This coupled with the fact I was not used to identifying and sharing my emotions anyway, meant I was not sharing my heart, my whole self with my wife. This creates an emotional barrier preventing us from feeling united and deeply connected.

It is also easy for lovemaking to become more functional, removing the intimacy from what is a such an emotionally bonding experience. Again, how we feel and what we are thinking, particularly during sex can make a difference in the way our body functions and the ability to conceive.

Do you feel an emotional connection to others?

"No, no-one understands what I am going through." Infertility can be a lonely place when friends and family don't truly understand what you are going through. This means that part of you is being kept from them, even your best friends, even your partner. This can create a barrier between you and them resulting in feeling isolated and impacting the emotional connection. You may be aware of how relationships and friendships have changed over time as they have had children and you are in a very different place to them.

Do you have a status in life (whatever it may be) that you value and that is acknowledged?

"No, I have lost my role and purpose in life, I have no status or purpose." Often people find their status and value comes from what they do, whether in some form of employment (paid or otherwise) or being a parent/homemaker. Infertility can change your priorities and values in life. Work no-longer becomes the source of your purpose. Deep down you believe your desire and purpose is to be a parent. Perhaps you have stopped work for a while to focus on your fertility, letting go of stress and changing your lifestyle – so again you have lost the status that work or your career brought. As time goes by you wonder what people think of you, not working, not at home to look after children. Caring for yourself over and above having a role can be necessary from time to time, however, society does not recognise or value that.

Are you achieving things in your life that you are proud of?

"No, the one thing I would be proud of I can't have." At the moment you probably cannot imagine achieving much as all your energy is being put into achieving the one thing you want – to have a baby.

Do you feel competent in at least one major area of your life?

"No, my body doesn't even do what it is supposed to do naturally." Infertility can knock your self-esteem sideways like a whack on the side of the head. Why can't your body do what it is designed and supposed to do naturally? You may feel incomplete, broken, not wholly a woman/man as a result.

Are you mentally and/or physically stretched in ways which give you a sense of meaning and purpose?

"I am mentally and physically exhausted not stretched but without any sense of meaning or purpose." Infertility can be physically and emotionally exhausting and a lot of people don't understand that. They think it is like not being able to have the job you want, you'll get over it, it'll pass. Or they think you are making too much of it and 'just need to relax' and it'll be fine.

Spend a moment now going through them asking yourself what you could do to improve it, even just one number higher.

13

❖

It's not what you do, it's why you do it

Whilst clearing out some paperwork I came across my test results from our fertility journey. I was interested in mapping out the dates of the tests/results to where we were on our journey as I made a number of life changes during it.

My first test result was disastrous. I went on a five-month programme to improve my fertility doing everything I believed could make a difference. Things like acupuncture, herbs, nutrition, not putting my phone in my pocket and wearing baggy pants! I was fully committed to the programme and was open to the possibility miracles could happen. I trust our doctor and he was optimistic an improvement could be made.

The next test five months later was actually marginally worse than the original. I didn't think that was possible!

At this point, I gave up trying as didn't believe I could do anything to improve my results. We were now in the hands of the clinic as far as I was concerned. It was all down to them from now. They were debating whether ICSI was an option for us given my results.

At the same time, I hit rock bottom emotionally.

This was a trigger for me to begin examining my life and why

I was unhappy. I thought having children would make me happy, give me a sense of fulfilment in life and now it looked like this was not going to happen.

In my reflection, I realised I felt like a victim in life. However, for the first time, I realised I had choices but I had to make them. I could choose to leave the job I didn't enjoy. I could choose to stop meeting other people's expectations and start living the life I wanted. I was going through the motions of life, doing the things I thought I should do, or the things that would please others. I wasn't living life to the full. I wasn't following my soul. Part of me was telling myself I wasn't allowed to be happy or have fun doing the things I really wanted to do. I was looking at life through a bunch of childhood thinking that was neither true nor serving me.

What I find interesting, but actually am not surprised about, is that we conceived naturally a few months after making these decisions and changes to my life. We weren't even trying because we thought there wasn't any point. Intrigued, I had another test to see what was going on and it was dramatically improved without me even trying to improve it.

Don't get me wrong, I still firmly believe in the power of things such as acupuncture, herbs, nutrition etc. on our physical and emotional well-being, including fertility. However in my personal experience, and that of my clients, our mind is incredibly powerful. The fear of treatments not working can cause a bigger impact on ourselves and our body than the benefits they bring.

In summary, it's not what we do, it's why we do it.

Whether it is taking daily temperatures, sticking to a nutrition plan, whatever it may be, if we have an underlying fear that it is not going to work then that fear could cause more damage than the positive effect of the actions we are taking. If we are scared we are not going to be successful because we haven't done absolutely everything that could work again we will be doing things out of fear and perhaps even finding them a chore or resenting it. This could be inadvertently feeding the fear of not succeeding.

You are far better off doing what you are inspired to do. If stopping something feels like a relief then stop it. It may not be forever, perhaps you or your body just needs a break for a while. It's about being in tune with your instinct, about what's right for you.

There is no formula for a successful pregnancy. What worked for one person may not work for someone else. No-one knows your body better than you. Not your fearful thinking self, your quiet instinct. Your intuition. Your gut feeling about what is right for you. What to do. What not to do.

It's not what we do, it's why we do it. What are you doing out of fear of not getting pregnant? What feels like a relief if you stopped doing it? Trust your intuition as to what is right for you at this moment in time.

On the same note, what are you not doing out of fear? What projects or life changes are you holding back on just in case you get pregnant? My clients have been holding back on all sorts of things out of fear of getting pregnant. Starting the new business, renovating the house, changing job. When is the right time? If you start creating the new business and you get pregnant will you care that it has to go on hold for a while?! When you put your life on hold and it stops flowing your body can stop flowing. The mind and body are one system.

So what are you doing out of fear that would feel a relief if you stopped?

What are you holding back doing out of fear that would feel life-giving if you did it?

14

❖

Striving v knowing you're OK

A lot of my clients have built success in areas of their lives, such as their career, relationships and other projects. Often they bring the mindset they applied to these successes to their fertility. It has brought success in the past so why not apply the same approach.

This approach in the past has been to have a clear goal, work hard, overcome the obstacles, stay focussed and you tend to achieve the thing you want.

They often felt a sense of being in control of their career, seeing the progress from their striving, however they find this way of being doesn't work with their fertility. For the first time in their life, they have an outcome they want to achieve but actually have no control over it. No matter how hard they work it doesn't always bring the desired outcome.

It can be very disconcerting not to feel in control of your fertility.

Their past successes have been built upon striving towards the goal. It can be stressful at times but that's OK as they know it comes with the territory and believe it'll be worth it.

When it comes to fertility, this approach often leads to obsessing about finding the thing that could make all the difference. Endless hours of research on the internet and reading of other people's stories on support forums trying to glean that one thing that made a difference you haven't yet tried or heard of.

However, this approach can actively be hindering your chances of getting pregnant.

Striving forward towards a goal is often fuelled by an 'outside-in' approach to life. Our thinking tells us that our happiness and well-being is dependent on circumstances on the outside. 'I'll be OK if...' Or 'I'll be OK when...'

It is very hard to control situations and circumstances on the outside and this can often lead to a very busy mind and lots of overthinking. Trying to control future outcomes with lots of 'what if' thinking. However, nothing can predict the future, not even our thinking.

When we begin to realise our sense of well-being, happiness and fulfilment comes from within and is not dependent on anything on the outside it is then we can begin to let go of this fear-based striving and find peace of mind.

In the workplace this enables us to have an uncluttered mind, to have clarity of mind that brings ideas and solutions and ultimately higher performance with less effort. We often think we need the striving or an element of pressure to perform at our best. However, in reality, no-one performs at their best under any amount of pressure. The old way of striving may have worked but I would argue it is possible to succeed with greater ease and well-being.

When it comes to fertility, the striving and the overthinking leads to stress and fear, which can actively reduce your chances of success. The mind and body are one system. The mind affecting the body, the body affecting the mind.

It's about holding the goal, whatever it is, lightly. Knowing you'd love to create that outcome but you don't need it for happiness and well-being because that comes from within. The outcome is a desire, not a need. On the other hand, you know you are OK in this moment. It is the creative energy between knowing we are OK now and having a goal held lightly that moves us forward towards it with ease and well-being. Which means we are far more likely to succeed.

Is what you are doing fuelled be fear or not succeeding or is it inspired action knowing whatever happens you will be OK? Because you will. You were born with innate well-being. You don't have to earn it or work your way towards it. It sure looks like that at times but that is the illusion of our thoughts and feelings.

Do you know whatever happens you are going to be OK?

There is a difference between knowing and KNOWING.

This is why I suggest focussing on Project You, not Project Baby. Once you truly know you are OK whatever happens, Project Baby tends to take more care of itself.

Part 2

How to get off the rollercoaster

15

❖

How to relax

The fertility emotional rollercoaster can be relentless. As well as being relentless, our base level of stress can often build up without us being aware. It becomes a new 'normal'. Just like boiling a frog. Apparently, if you put a frog in boiling water it will jump out. However, if you put it in cold water and put it on to boil it will stay in the water until the water boils and it dies (who found that out, and why?!). We often don't realise how much stress we are carrying mentally and physically.

This journey is connecting you to your innate well-being through understanding what's creating our human experience and re-connecting to our true sense of self. It's about not relying on 'tools and techniques' to keep you together. Relying on techniques can be hard work as it can be fighting Thought with Thought. It rarely ends well!

That said, whilst you are on this journey of understanding having some things that help you get out of the pot of boiling water, even for just a short time, can make a huge difference to your well-being and state of mind. It can help you begin to see things with greater clarity and perspective in the moment, waking you up from the trance of Outside-In Thought.

So, how do you relax? I've met plenty of clients who say they don't do anything to relax. Who can't sit and do nothing, their thinking is going so quickly their mind needs constant stimulation, e.g. have to have the TV or radio on when in the house on their own, they don't like silence. It's often a sign of a habitual busy mind.

The first thing to acknowledge is that everyone is different and we don't all find the same thing relaxing. Some people find cooking relaxing. Not me (unless it is a recipe I know well!). The founder of Cognitive Hypnotherapy, Trevor Silvester, who trained me had an example of this when he first qualified as a hypnotherapist. He was taught to relax people by getting them to imagine they were walking along a beach. One of his first clients burst into tears as he did this with her as she has just broken up from her fiancé whilst walking along a beach! This is the seed sown for developing Cognitive Hypnotherapy which works with each person's 'model of the world' rather than assuming one thing works for everyone. So give yourself permission to do what you find relaxing and not what you think you 'should' do.

In general, we relax when we get out of our heads and come back to the present moment, reconnecting with our body and our environment. Anything that can help you do this can help you relax, whether going for a walk in nature, doing some yoga or just sitting and focussing on your breath. They all work by doing the same thing; Waking you up from the trance you are in. Breaking the trance created by all your thinking in your head about the future and past and bringing you back to the here and now. Even a hot bath does this because it helps you use your senses to feel what you are feeling in the moment, not feeling what you are thinking is going to happen over the next few weeks and months.

Here are two techniques I often teach clients to help them break the trance of fear, sadness or anger and come back to the here and now and their emotional resilience and well-being.

3–5 Breathing

This is a profoundly simple but effective relaxation breathing exercise that you can use any time, any place, anywhere and no-one will know you are doing it!

This technique utilises a natural biological relaxation process as well as bringing your mind to the present moment. It forces your out breathe to be longer than your in breathe. When you do this you utilise more carbon dioxide in the breath. Carbon dioxide is a natural biological relaxant. It is why when someone hyperventilates you often see them breathing into a paper bag. They are recirculating their breath and taking in more carbon dioxide.

- Simply concentrate on your breathing and count from 1-3 as you breathe in and from 1-5 as you exhale.
- You can count out loud or in your head but if possible out loud can make it more effective.
- It doesn't need to be big breaths, just normal relaxed breathing adjusting the pace of the counting to your breath.
- After 10-15 breaths you may start to notice how much more relaxed you're beginning to feel.
- If your mind wanders just bring it gently back to your breath.

Dropthrough

This is a way of letting go of a feeling you feel stuck in and to regain a sense of peace of mind and emotional well-being.

- When you are feeling an emotion you want to let go of, perhaps anxiety, sadness, grief, etc. name the emotion and then take a deep breath in. As you breathe out imagine falling through, or dropping through that emotion. Like falling through a trap door. Imagine dropping through the emotion and you will find another emotion underneath it. There is always an emotion under an emotion.

- Name this new one and then repeat. Take a deep breath and drop through that feeling.

- Keep doing this until you get to a place of no feeling. Some people experience it as a cloud, or void or bubble. Rest in this place for a little while. Enjoy the feeling of it.

- Then when you are ready to take another deep breath in and drop through that place and you will come to a positive emotion (such as peace, hope, love). Enjoy this place and breathe it in.

- Do not drop through any further as you may find yourself going full circle! In which case keep going back round to the positive emotion.

So play with ways you find relaxing to help you find respite from the emotional rollercoaster.

As we go through this journey together we shall be focussing on a fresh understanding of what is creating your experience moment to moment. This gives you a new perspective of yourself and life rather than having to keep fighting the tide of emotions with tools and techniques. The difference can be between trying to use armband tools to stay afloat and realising you float. You can lie on your back and enjoy the gentle bobbing of the waves knowing that wherever the tide takes you, you are OK.

16

❖

The grand illusion

There are three misunderstandings that prevent us from having peace of mind regardless of what's happening in life, whether the pain of infertility or something else. I want to introduce them to you here but we shall be exploring each one in more detail over this section of the book and seeing how they play out in everyday life.

The first is a misunderstanding of the nature of Thought. I'm using Thought with a capital T for a reason because I want to distinguish between Thought and the cognitive thinking in our head. Here I'm referring to what creates our perception of reality. It's the layer between the outside world and human experience. It creates every perceptual experience we have. What we see, taste, feel, etc. Thought doesn't create our circumstances but creates our experience of them.

We cannot control Thought. You couldn't choose your next Thought even if you wanted to. Thought is personal in the way that your flavour of habitual Thought is personal to you, shaped by your upbringing, your interpretation of situations etc. over the years. However, it is in-personal by the fact you don't choose your next Thought. Everything we experience is Thought. Anger, fear, judgement, love, peace, joy. All thought. Thought is also always moving to peace of mind and clarity if we allow it. That's our default state of mind. It may not be our learned habitual state, but when we stop trying to be OK and stop interfering with the system it settles back to a place of clarity and perspective.

The second misunderstanding is a misunderstanding of what creates our experience. As we have already begun exploring in the previous section nothing makes us feel anything. It is our perception of the situation that we are experiencing. We are experiencing everything behind the veil of Thought. Thought is neutral until it comes into our consciousness and creates our experience. The illusion is that it looks and feels like this experience is coming from the outside world – our situation, the past or the future. It looks like our experience works Outside-In but it only works one way, Inside-Out.

It is like watching a film. The best films we enjoy are the ones where at times we forget it's a film. We are so absorbed in the acting, the special-effects and the directorship we spend times forgetting it is not real. Watching the films we least enjoy we are completely disengaged. Watching like a critic. Thinking of other films we have seen the actors in. Not seduced by the acting, special-effects and directorship. Our mind is the same. We get seduced by Thoughts coming alive in our consciousness. It is so plausible and realistic we forget it's not real. It has the best special-effects department in the world, our emotions. How many times do we get caught up worrying about something only to find the next day we were worried about nothing. We even ask ourselves 'what was I thinking?'. Our experience only works one way. Inside-out.

The third misunderstanding is a misunderstanding of where our well-being comes from. Outside-in Thought believes our psychological well-being is dependent on something external to us. For example, 'I'm OK if people think I'm OK'. 'I'm OK if I have enough money in the bank.' This is based on the illusion that something on the outside can make us feel something on the inside. There are plenty of people who have more money than they know what to do with who are at peace and happy. Likewise, there are people who have more money than they know what to do with who are still unhappy. There are plenty of people on the bread-line who are content. And there are plenty of people on the bread-line who are stressed and unhappy.

We are born with innate well-being. Complete psychological well-being. Physically our body is always trying to restore back to health. If you cut yourself your body heals. If you break a bone your body knits them back together. This is in the context of us degrading over time with age but within that context, your body is always trying to restore back to health. Even with an extreme like cancer, your body is trying to dispel the foreign body. The same is true for our psychological health. Our default state is clarity, peace, and perspective.

There is an energy behind the life that enables life to hang together. That enables shoal of fish to swim together and know what to do. That enables a cut to heal itself. There is a formless energy behind life that we are never going to understand in our human form. This formless energy is whatever God, life, the universe, mother nature is for you. It is loving, creative and divine. We are made of that energy, we are part of that energy. It doesn't make anything defective. It doesn't make anything that needs to prove itself. When we have a quiet mind it is this energy we are connecting with. Our soul is made of it, part of it. We are spiritual beings having a human experience. Our true self is the observer of this experience. Our true self knows we are OK whatever we are experiencing in this world of form. This energy is the potential behind life that enables any experience.

To summarise these three aspects of our human experience. Our mind works like an old film projector. Thought is the reel of film. On its own it is neutral. It doesn't really create much of a human experience. The projector is our consciousness. This is where Thought comes alive and creates a human experience. Thought is neutral until we give it our attention and it comes into our consciousness. Creating an illusion so plausible and believable we forget it's not real. And the energy behind life is the electricity the projector is plugged into. It's the potential to have any experience.

This can be a big concept to grasp and we shall be unpacking it over this section of the book to see how the more you understand these principles behind our human experience the easier it is for you to get off the emotional rollercoaster and find greater peace, resilience and innate well-being.

17

❖

We are built for reality

"You are braver than you believe, stronger than you seem and smarter than you think." A. A. Milne.

On our fertility journey there were times I thought I didn't have the strength to carry on. To continue going through the motions of life surrounded by reminders of what I hadn't got and wanted the most in the world.

I once had a conversation with a lady who lost her 3 year old son to cancer. I asked if someone told her she was going to experience that what would her reaction have been. She said she would have said there is no way she could cope with something like that, it would finish her. Here she was on the other side of it. She'd found inner strength and resilience she never knew she had amongst the sheer grief and pain.

Our human operating system is designed for reality. We have evolved over millions of years and there is a built-in quality-check nature has provided to ensure we are optimised for thriving in reality. This quality-check has been applied to every one of your ancestors going back millions of years. Whether they were strong enough, fit enough, resilient enough, brave enough, wise enough to survive and pass on their genes to the next generation. So you being the product of all that means that your genes have passed those tests hundreds of thousands of times!

We have an innate capability for clarity, resilience, creativity, direction, wisdom, intuition amongst others. Everything we need to thrive in this moment, in reality, is built within us.

Traditionally we hunted and gathered. You couldn't hunt and gather successfully without being fully present. If you were not present to reality you would either not see the berries you needed or your risk of being attacked by a sabretooth tiger! We have everything we need to thrive in this moment.

This human operating system has been finely tuned over millions of years. It is this operating system that enables a baby to move from a gravity free floating environment to learning to feed, find its hands and feet, learn to walk and learn to talk. All without any flashcards or external tuition. We don't teach a baby to do those things, it comes from within them. They learn what they need to survive and thrive in reality.

A toddler doesn't worry about tomorrow or get hung up about yesterday. A toddler doesn't bear grudges. Toddlers spend far more time in the here and now than most adults who are more contaminated by Outside-In thinking. Little children don't worry about whether they are good enough, attractive enough, what may or may not happen in the future or hold on to what happened in the past.

Toddlers are far more aware of our innate well-being. They don't question their psychological well-being because they are far more aware of this inbuilt operating system that knows they are OK and takes one moment at a time. Yes, they are still human and occasionally get caught up in stories about the future. They have tantrums. Telling themselves that their life is not worth living because they cannot have a sweet in that moment! But then they go back to being in the moment and they settle back to being calm and grounded as if it never happened.

I'll never forget the day our dog had to be put down out of

the blue. My son was six at the time. I've never seen him cry so hard and be so upset. But then it was like flicking a switch. He stopped and went back to being OK. He cried a little later on but again went back to being OK. Is it that he didn't care much about the dog? Far from it. They were thick as thieves. For me, this is an example of our innate capacity of well-being, part of our inbuilt operating system that gives us all we need to deal with reality.

People who are worried about losing their job are more anxious about the thought of losing than if it actually happened. When it happens, it's not what they choose but they get on with it. They are in reality and the resources they need to deal with it show up, when we are in reality and not our future thinking la la land.

Just like little children, our human operating system is comfortable with the unknown. Knowing our innate-well-being is not dependant on anything external, anything happening in the past, present or future. It's core to our operating system. Knowing this, children are comfortable with the unknown, with not knowing. This brings them a sense of wonder to life. Many adults could benefit from reconnecting with this sense of wonder and possibility.

When we think about the future we tend to imagine worse-case scenarios and all our resources that enable us to thrive in the moment are not present. We are not designed for our future la la land imagination of the future. We are designed for reality. So when we think about the future our wisdom is not present. Our resourcefulness is not present. No wonder it can look scary or feel as if we can't cope when we think about a future scenario. Our wisdom shows up in the moment when we need it. This is why events are usually never as bad as we imagine them to be.

Our innate operating system has everything we need in this moment. Clarity, perspective, intuition, well-being, insights, creativity, connection. You don't have to do anything to obtain these. Trying to think your way to these capacities is like trying to grab a feather. It alludes you. They come to you naturally in the moment. This is why the days you feel happiest and most alive are when you are just being. You haven't done anything to get into that state, you drop into it when your Outside-In thinking collapses and you come back to reality.

18

❖

Responding to feelings

A friend of mine is going through a marriage breakdown. His wife is leaving him. He is devastated. However, he's not actually feeling the pain of it. He's in denial. Part of him thinks if he doesn't feel it he doesn't have to face the reality of the situation. It reminded me that as a rule of thumb there are three ways we can respond to an emotion.

One way is to simply avoid it as my friend is doing. We can be aware of it lurking in the background, wanting to rise up and flood our system. However, another part of us is resisting it for many reasons. Perhaps we think if we feel the emotion such as distress, fear or anger we judge ourselves or our life as failures. We think if we feel the emotion we become powerless, a victim to the situation that is causing the feeling.

When I was first self-employed I used to be fearful about earning enough money. I thought if I entertained the fear it would mean it was true. I wasn't going to earn enough money or I wasn't good enough at doing what I was doing to earn enough money. The result was an ongoing battle with background fear and being fearful of the fact it was there and what it 'meant'.

Another reason for resisting feelings can be a belief that if we feel the emotion we may fall into it and never come out. I had a client, Dan, who had been depressed for many years. Working together he reconnected to his innate well-being. It was like he was transformed. Back to his happy-go-lucky self. And then something happened that triggered a bunch of fearful thinking and he started to feel down again. However what made it worse was the fear of going back to how he was. He thought if he felt down it would be a one-way ticket back to being depressed for a long time.

This approach of avoidance doesn't serve us. It is fighting the reality of our human experience in the moment and actually weakens us rather than empowers us. It is based on the belief that we are only OK if we feel OK. It goes back to that misunderstanding of where our well-being comes from. Outside-In Thought believes that we are only OK if we feel OK so if we don't feel OK there we're not OK. When Dan saw this playing out and allowed himself to feel whatever he is feeling knowing underneath his human experience he's still OK it passed so much quicker than he could imagine and was back to his innate happy self.

Another approach to an emotion is to collapse into it. This is sometimes referred to as emotional hijacking. The emotion hijacks our sense of perspective and clarity. Again we become a victim, judging that things should be different, blaming ourselves or others (even subconsciously) and losing perspective and clarity in the moment.

When we collapse into an emotion we can become stressed, defensive, irritable. We are subconsciously telling ourselves it is a 'bad' thing that we are feeling this, that it means something is 'wrong' and we feel powerless to change it or blame the situation or others for causing it. I can collapse into an emotion of fear and then end up being grumpy to be around. I've collapsed and ended up taking it out on others or 'life' unconsciously.

I've noticed this physically as well. When I am resisting reality on a run, getting annoyed about the rain or wind my head goes down, my shoulders come forward, the top of my body collapses physically.

There is a third way. It is possible to feel an emotion such as anger or fear and stay open to it. For your heart to stay open. To feel it without judgment or evaluation. Without judging you or the situation as good, bad, right or wrong or what it means for you or the future. It is what it is in this moment. To feel emotions is called being human! We can feel an emotion but still know we are OK. Knowing it is a Thought-created experience allows us to stay open in it.

When my father died I felt a deep sense of grief, but I still knew I was going to be OK. It wasn't telling me anything about the future, it wasn't telling me that life was never going to be as good without him because nothing can predict the future. Also as humans happiness and well-being come from within us, we are not dependant on anything on the outside for psychological well-being. I still felt devastated. But it allowed me to feel the grief but keep my heart open to it instead of running from it or even getting so lost in it that it becomes sorrow.

When I am running and allowing the weather to be whatever it is, without resistance or judgement my head is up and I am upright. Before I know it I forget to think about it and it's no longer in my awareness. When I am angry with my wife and I stay open it keeps us in a conversation that is fighting for clarification and getting back to unity rather than collapsing in to the emotion and either shutting down or fighting to be right (don't get me wrong that happens as well, I am not the perfect husband!).

The bottom line is the less we care how we are feeling because we know the true source of our well-being and that we are living in a Thought created experience, the more we feel happy, content and grounded. That's because it's our default state of mind as humans. It may not be our habitual state but when we stop interfering with the system we spent more time in our default.

It's never the feeling that's the problem, it's our feelings about our feeling. Our anxiety about being anxious. The more we allow feelings, notice them but don't go beyond noticing, they have less impact on our consciousness and pass more quickly than you imagine.

Embrace your humanness knowing your feelings are not a reflection on life or you. It will soon pass as Thought (and thus emotion) comes and goes like clouds on a breeze. Knowing you have what you need to deal with whatever shows up in reality. You are not the clouds, you are the sky.

When you feel the pain of this journey don't be scared of it. You've got what it takes to ride the storm. Don't resist it. Don't resent it. You may not feel it but you are stronger than feelings. Allow it and you may be surprised how quickly it passes and a fresh state of mind and resourcefulness follow behind it.

19

Role of thinking

If I asked you to take a magic pill that meant you would never think again would you take it?

99% of people I ask that question say no. They can perhaps see they have some unhelpful or negative thinking, or that perhaps at times they overthink. They would like to let go of those habits, but in general, they think they need their thinking.

Think about the times you have been most content in life. Perhaps times with loved ones or appreciating a scene in nature. How much is on your mind in those times? Most people recognise not a lot. That is a moment of being.

Think of times when you feel like you're on fire. Perhaps at work performing brilliantly and life feels effortless. In a state of flow. Again how much is on your mind at these times? Usually not a lot. We are still making decisions but they are more instinctive.

You see we think we need our thinking but actually, we perform our best in a more content state with less on our minds. When we think we need our thinking we often stop discerning between Outside-In Thought and Inside-Out Thought. This can leave us chasing our tail trying to think our way back to peace and clarity.

So why do we have Outside-In thinking if it doesn't serve us? Well, we probably need it to survive and be in this physical word.

We need it to protect us from physical danger. But we tend to unnecessarily apply it to psychological well-being.

We come into the world with everything we need psychologically: with innate well-being, contentment and peace of mind. When was the last time you looked at a baby and thought they weren't complete, perfect? Toddlers spend most of their time just 'being', content in the moment. It makes sense, given we are human 'beings'.

But then life happens. Life is a contact sport. We live in a world that thinks it works Outside-In. We had parents that probably thought it worked Outside-In. I know mine did. My Mum was convinced I would be more OK with better exam results and a job with a final salary pension. Don't get me wrong there is nothing wrong with getting good exam results but our psychological well-being is not dependant on them or anything. Our soul's desire inspires our fulfilment. That may involve a desire for a specific career and we know good grades will help make that happen. But nothing makes us happy or secure, no job or purchase (contrary to what the adverts say). What makes us feel happy and secure is living connected to our soul, living from the Inside-Out.

Whether through parenting, schooling or being in society generally, we start to get caught into Outside-In Thought.

Neuroscientist Paul D. MacLean formulated a model of the brain in the 1960s based on three distinct structures of the brain as part of its evolution. The oldest most primitive part of our brain is the reptilian brain. It is at the top of the spinal cord at the base of the brain. Its function is that of reptiles; to find food and to stay alive.

The next evolutionary part of the brain is the mammalian brain, the limbic system often referred to as the emotional brain.

It wants to keep us safe and secure and be aware of danger. Mammals hunt and gather in tribes and packs. They want to be part of the pack as their survival is dependant on being part of the pack. This part of our brain wants to be loved.

Then there is the human brain. The cortex that gives humans the ability of lateral thinking, creativity and abstract thought.

It's the mammalian brain, the emotional brain that wants to be loved that controls the flight or fight response we explored in the last section. It thinks our survival is dependant on the pack staying together and our position in the pack being secure.

Growing up in this pack is more often than not the family unit but could be friendship circles or other perceived tribes/groups. If as a child we think in some way that the pack is not secure, perhaps parents arguing, or our position in the pack is not secure (we don't feel unconditional love) we can think subconsciously our survival is under threat. We begin to think we need to think to create a feeling of security. To keep the pack together or ensure we are loved and wanted within it.

My mum suffered from anxiety. She was a very strict schoolteacher and was like that at home. I know 100% my mum loved me unconditionally. I know 100% everything she did was motivated by love and she did the best she could with the resources she had available, including our own limiting thoughts and beliefs. As adults, we can look back and see things with emotional intelligence. As children, we don't see it that way or experience it that way. As children, we think our parents or caregivers or adults around us are perfect. We can't imagine them having their 'stuff' or problems.

As a child when I behaved in a way that pleased my mum she was happy and I felt more loved. And if I didn't she was angry I didn't feel loved. I learned the rules pretty quickly. Over time habitually I began to believe 'I'm OK if she's OK'. I started thinking life worked Outside-In. I did what I did to feel more loved and secure.

Our Outside-In thinking starts in all innocence, and properly served us in some way as a child, but continues out of habit. It can become the filter of Thought we see life through without being aware we are looking through a filter.

To make sense of the present moment, our mind goes back into the past to look for a match of information. For example, how would you know a chair is safe to sit on unless you've seen a chair before? Fear and worry are all about future thinking perhaps based on past experience.

I always I thought I was a worrier, I thought it was my 'personality type'. My mum was a worrier, I'm a worrier. But that's not who I am. We are not born worriers. We are born with an innate well-being, peace of mind. I lived in an environment where things were quite unpredictable, I was constantly second-guessing outcomes of my behaviour to try and ensure life was more peaceful and positive, that ultimately I felt more loved. Now if I feel stressed and pressurised I know it's nothing to do with what I'm doing in the moment, has nothing to do with my workload of that day – it is habitual Thought from the past. Previously I would have thought I needed to work longer or harder to clear my to-do list, as the feeling of stress was telling me that not doing so meant something bad would happen whether that would be my practice failing or missing out on 'the' opportunity to be the success I wanted to be.

It is this thinking we bring to our fertility journey. Our day to day experiences on our fertility journey is not about fertility. It is Thought habits we have about life and about ourselves that we bring and apply to our situation and future.

A client, Joanna, 38 had four failed IVF cycles before she worked with me. We quickly identified that the thinking behind her fear of not getting pregnant was all to do with validation. Fear of not being good enough. She could see how this has been playing out in her life for as long as she can remember but was unaware that it was underpinning her fear of not getting pregnant. Fear leads to stress. Fear holds us back. It was Thought that was creating this.

Looking back, when has your instinct ever let you down? When we look back we can see it hasn't. Your instinct is your wisdom. It includes your knowledge, your life experience and your intellect. Just without the contamination of Outside-In Thought.

If you could trust your instinct in this moment, your inner wisdom, your gut, what does it tell you about your fertility journey?

20

Nature of Thought

I am using the word Thought with a capital T to distinguish between conscious thoughts we have in our head (our ability to think) and the ability to create a perceptual reality. Thought is the source of all our experiences in life as well as the source of thoughts and perceptions that come in to our consciousness throughout the day.

So if Thought creates our experience and we spend a lot of time trying to manage our experience, for example avoiding stress, we spend a lot of time managing or fighting the effects of Thought.

I want to explore the nature of Thought. To move further up-stream away from the engineering of Thought, the impact it has on our experience, to look at the physics of Thought as a concept.

A dog chases its tail because it misunderstands the nature of a tail. As soon as a dog understands the tail is part of the dog it stops chasing it. The more we understand the true nature of thought we stop chasing it, stop trying to think a way back to peace, perspective, and clarity.

Thought is the layer between this world of form and our soul's formless experience of it. Everything we experience comes from Thought. Even our experience of pain comes from Thought. The source of the pain may be an exposed nerve or broken bone but the experience of the pain is Thought. Sometimes it's in our consciousness and it's agony, at other times we are not so aware of it.

Thought is self-correcting. Left to its own devices it settles to a place of clarity and perspective. It's always moving back to our innate Inside-Out well-being uncontaminated by Outside-In Thought. It is like a glitter ball, the more we shake it, the more we try to get back to peace and clarity the more we are putting energy into it, thinking about our experience rather than allowing it, a state of mind where it settles on its own.

The thing is, Outside-In thinking is very plausible, realistic and persuasive. It creates is an illusion of reality, that in some way our psychological well-being is dependant on something external to us. It provides all the evidence from the past to back it up which means, more easily than we like, we fall for it and go on a journey with it.

It's like a magic trick. I have a friend who does close-up magic. I know it is a trick, sleight of hand. Even though I know it's a trick he gets me every time! It's mesmerising.

It's the same with Thought. We fall for it, and we will continue to do so from time to time because it's called being human. However, the more we understand the true nature of Thought and the principles behind our human experience the less we get tricked by it. If my friend shows me how the trick is done and I then watch him do it on someone else I can't believe I didn't see through the illusion when he did it with me originally.

Understanding the principles behind our human experience helps us to get tricked by Outside-In Thought less and less. As a consequence, we spend more time grounded in the present moment, connected to our innate well-being and resourcefulness for life.

Another thing about Thought is that all Thoughts is equal. We can believe some Thought is more important than other

Thought. That some need to be listened to more than others. A colleague of mine's two-year-old girl wanted a sweet but he said no for various reasons. As toddlers sometimes do, she had a tantrum about the fact she couldn't have a sweet. His initial thought was 'hey missy, if you get this worked up about having a sweet wait until you have to worry about paying your bills etc.'. Because that's what got him worked up.

Then he had an insight. Her reality at that moment was no different to when he gets caught up worrying about paying the bills. Both are Inside-Out illusions. Both are creating their 'reality' in that moment. Trying to tell his two year old that having a sweet wasn't that important was futile because her reality in that moment was that it was. When he got worked up about paying his bills trying to tell him that whatever happens he will be OK is futile, he's caught up in the Outside-In illusion. That's his reality in that moment.

Of course not paying the bills has a bigger consequence than not having a sweet! However, regardless of the consequence, nothing can make us feel anything. Whether you can pay the bills doesn't make you feel anything. There are people who are on the breadline and in debt and content. There are people in that situation who are very much not at peace. It's not the circumstances, it's our thinking about it that creates the experience. It only works one way regardless of the circumstances.

His thinking about paying the bills was not more important than her thinking about the sweet. Both were creating their reality in that moment. Both had taken them Outside-In.

I used to think Thought was the bad stuff. My (over) thinking was creating my fear, anxiety and feeling of insecurity. I used to resent Thought. I had a massive insight one day when I realised everything is Thought. Everything we experience, whether love, peace and joy; or fear, anger and jealousy.

I had Outside-In thinking, perhaps fear, and then resentful thinking about my fearful thinking. I was just adding more and more to it, getting more and more caught up in the Outside-In experience.

Thought is like a conveyor belt. There are Thoughts of all shapes and sizes. It's spontaneous. We can't choose the next Thought. It's personal in that the typical or habitual flavour of Thought we tend to have is dependant on our upbringing and our experiences in life that have shaped our perception of ourselves and life.

In the 1980s there was a game show called The Generation Game. At the end of the show the finalist sat in front of a conveyor belt on which a stream of prizes came past. At the end all the prizes they could remember they got to keep. When we resent our thinking, or resist it, or even wish we weren't having it, we are going on a journey with a particular train of Thought. This prevents new fresh Inside-Out Thought coming through. It stops the self-correcting system kick in.

Thought is impersonal in the fact you cannot choose your next Thought even if you wanted to. We are not thinking beings. We are beings that have Thought.

All your Thought about whether you will get pregnant or not, about the unfairness of the situation, the fear of not being the mother you want to be is actually spontaneous Thought. You cannot control it. You cannot choose to stop it. Step back and see how it is a stream of consciousness, a conveyor belt of experiences and that left to its own devices moves to peace and clarity all on its own. Stop trying to manage your state of mind, thinking you need to 'think positive'. Allow the conveyor belt of thought to find its own way back to your innate well-being, resilience and clarity. You are not your thinking, you are the observer of all your thinking. The more we see this the less embroiled we get in to Thought that just stops fresh Thought coming in to our awareness.

21

Perception v reality

My heart started to race, everything was in the car. And now it had gone. The car was not where I left it. I had been travelling home after being away so everything from clothes to my laptop was in the car. Interestingly I was more worried about the laptop than the car!

I've never had a car stolen before; all I was thinking was the hassle, expense, and frustration. Just a moment ago I was enjoying the sunshine and looking forward to the weekend. Now I was in a blind panic filled with anger, frustration, and fear of how I was going to cope without my laptop and all the information on it (unusually and foolishly the backup was in the laptop bag!).

As I looked at the space where my car had been parked behind the white van where I'd left it, there was now a smaller car in the bigger space. Someone had clearly parked in the space created by my car being stolen. How could it have happened in broad daylight with loads of people milling around? It wasn't an area I was very familiar with and I looked further up the road questioning whether it was possible that I had parked further down the road. The walk back to the car did seem quicker than going, but doesn't it always?

As I looked down the road I saw a roundabout and absolutely knew I hadn't walked across it. I also couldn't place where cars could park beyond the roundabout. I knew I had to call the police to report the car stolen but I did not want to make the call, I did not want to believe what was happening.

I decided to walk further down the road just to make 100% sure I hadn't made a mistake. As I walked down the unfamiliar road, I rounded a bend. There was another white van and with my car parked behind it, just as I'd left it!

The relief was overwhelming. As I drove off it all started to come back to me. I was attending a busy event. I remembered that after I parked the car and continued to the event on foot I made a phone call and was just following the crowd without really paying attention to my surroundings. So I realised I had walked across the roundabout that only moments before I was totally convinced I hadn't.

At that moment my reality was my car had been stolen and I was feeling the repercussions of that. About calling the police. This is how we live life. We live life through our perception of reality. Perception drives feelings. Perception drives behaviour.

I once heard George Pransky share a story that he had gone camping with his wife and another couple one summer's weekend. They drove to a national park to camp in the forest. When they got set up he said to his friend they'd better go and collect some firewood so they can build a fire and get cooking. His friend said they would do that but there was plenty of time and no hurry. George got a little agitated and said that it was getting late and they didn't want to be cooking in the dark so they'd better go now. They went off and collected the wood and built a fire. George then said to his wife, Linda, that they'd better get cooking as it was getting late. Again she said to him that there was plenty of time and to relax. Once again George got agitated and said it was getting late and they didn't want to be cooking in the dark so they'd better get cooking. Linda said to George,

'George it's only 4 o'clock in the afternoon, you've still got your sunglasses on!'

George had left his sunglasses on from the drive in the sunshine. They were now in the forest and the sun was starting to go down. The moment she said that he realised what was creating his experience wasn't what he thought it was his whole experience shifted, even before he took his sunglasses off! The more we see what is creating our experience we can realise it's not what we think it is, it's not circumstances but Thought in this moment, we can stop going on a journey of Thought and come back to reality where we have clarity, perspective and resourcefulness.

Just as we create our own perception of reality through Thought so does everyone else. There were 7 million perceptions of reality out there. When a number of people tend to think the same they think it is reality. It just means a lot of people think the same. If 100% of our experience comes from our perception of reality, what is reality? Everyone is experiencing their perception of life.

If we think there is one 'right' way of seeing things we can get easily frustrated or annoyed if people don't think the same as us. We can think our way of thinking is right and theirs is wrong. Both are perceptions created by Thought. Neither is right or wrong, good or bad. They just are what they are. The more we see everyone is living in the experience of thought, separate realities at this moment, we have the ability to have more compassion and understanding for others. We judge their behaviour less and can see it is coming from their reality at that moment which makes sense to them as it's created by Thought in the moment.

A lot of the clients I see are in some way worried about what people think of them. Perhaps they are scared of being judged or not meeting others' expectations. Or scared they won't think

well of them. The more we can see that we live in separate realities, that their thinking is just their thinking, not truth or reality,
we can care less about what the content of it is. Not only is it
Thought in the moment, shaped by their stuff, their stories, limiting beliefs and fears, but it doesn't have the power to make you
feel anything. It's your Thought about what they may be thinking
that is creating your experience. The reality is you are OK with
who you are regardless of what others think.

I can make so many assumptions about life and the future
that look so plausible and believable but the truth is nothing can
predict the future, not even your thinking. Fear of not getting
pregnant is future thinking. It looks so believable in times of low
mood. 100% of your experience is Thought in the moment, not
reality. The more you see that the less you get caught up on the
train of Thought that takes you to fearful places.

22

❖

What the thinker thinks, the prover proves

We were once staying in a quiet residential town in northern California. We were on a health retreat. Our host encouraged us to get out every morning and go for a walk. Having a dog back home, we were very much used to doing that and enjoyed our morning walks. However, our host warned us that it was not a friendly neighbourhood. She said the people that live there were suspicious of each other so don't be surprised if people were not friendly.

I know we were the novelty being the Brits in a non-touristy residential area of America, however, our experience of the locals was the opposite of her description. Meeting the same people each morning walking their dogs over the days the conversations became longer. Invitations to meals were offered. Home-grown produce from their gardens given. I was even invited to a men's breakfast club where a group of friends had met every single day for the past 30 years to have breakfast together before they start their day. Our host was shocked. She started coming out on the walks with us to see what we were doing!

The more time we spent with our host the more her negative and fearful mindset became apparent. She saw what she wanted to see. So that was the experience she got.

There's a lovely story I've heard George Pransky share. Imagine a man goes to pay for his fuel at a petrol station. He asked the man behind the counter 'What are the people like in this area? We are thinking of moving up here from down south'. The server responds by asking him what they are like where he comes from. The man replies, 'Oh they are not very friendly at all, very distrusting of each other'. The server says 'You'll find the people around here are just like that'. The man responds 'Thank you so much for the heads up. You've saved us a lot of hassle, we'll look elsewhere'.

A little while later another man comes to pay for his fuel. He asked the man behind the counter, 'What are the people like in this area? We are thinking of moving down here from up north'. Again the server responds by asking him what they are like where he comes from. The man replies 'They are really friendly, such a great sense of community. We love it there but we need to move because of work'. Again the server says, 'You'll find the people around here are just like that'. The man responds 'That's great, we shall look forward to settling in the area'.

There is a phrase called Orr's Law. 'What the thinker thinks, the prover proves'. We have a thinker part of us and a prover part of us. The prover looks for all the evidence to back up our thinking. We dismiss anything to the contrary. Let me explain how it works.

When we take in information through our senses our conscious mind cannot take in everything, it would result in brain overload! Our unconscious mind takes it all in but what we are consciously aware of is far less than that.

This huge volume of information from our senses (circa 2 million bits of information/second) needs to be filtered down to something more manageable. The filters used to do this are shaped by our thoughts, beliefs and values (aka Thought) and they do one of three things. They either distort, generalise or delete information coming in through the senses. The resulting information you receive in your mind is your 'model of the world'.

It is your take on life, experience and situations. This is why you might find yourself reminiscing with friends and family about past events and you all have a different memory of it. You all had a very different experience of it at the time which is going to shape your memories.

Have you wondered why people do things that you think is just so illogical? Or perhaps wonder why they do things the particular way they do which again seems completely illogical to you?

Whilst staying with my father-in-law I was baffled at how he organised things in his house. When I enquired as to why he kept cold remedy with the jam in the kitchen but the rest of his medicines elsewhere he said the reason was it was the medicine he uses most so it was somewhere convenient to get to. This made me wonder about how often he got colds, however I was pleased to find out he actually wasn't needing it as frequently as he put jam on his toast!

To him, it was completely logical, in his model of the world. To me, it was illogical and getting cold remedy from the bathroom cabinet didn't seem too arduous!

Let me give you another example. We all lose our keys or phone from time to time. When looking for your keys how many times do you find them in a place where you looked twice? It's amazing, isn't it? Why didn't we see them the first time?

When you are looking for your keys you are probably telling yourself, 'I can't find my keys…where are my keys? I can't find my keys,' etc. Your unconscious mind does not want to make a liar of you so what happens? It deletes the keys from your vision. It is called negative hallucination in the trade. You simply don't see them. Next time you lose your keys tell yourself over and over 'I can find my keys' and you may be surprised how much more quickly you find them.

There are, no doubt, times where all you can see around you are pregnant women, or couples cooing over a newborn baby. It's tough, isn't it? I remember the pain of seeing a father with their young children. The fact you see so many may be partly due to a thought process that 'everyone is having babies except me'. Your unconscious mind will then go and look for the evidence to back that up. You will literally see more and more babies/pregnant women as a result of this.

Be mindful of the stories creating the lens you are experiencing life and your fertility journey through.

23

Imagination

I can do worry big time. I can convince myself something bad is going to happen. I find all the reasons why I need to believe it. It's so convincing to me I can't believe others can't see it. I could never imagine us being happy without children. For me it was the only way we would be truly happy. It was fact as far as I was concerned.

Worry is the misuse of imagination. But what do I mean by imagination? I think most people would say imagination is thinking of something that is made up, perhaps even unrealistic. Maybe something like winning the lottery or telling our boss exactly what we really think of them!

I could imagine flying (if I could pick a super-power it would definitely be flying!) through the sky, soaring like an eagle. That's imagination. Or I could imagine my car turning in to a helicopter and lifting me out of the traffic jam and flying on to my destination. That's also clearly imagination. Both unrealistic and beyond reality.

I could imagine big scary monsters, however I wouldn't be frightened as I know it is my imagination. I know it's unrealistic.

Unconsciously assuming this definition of imagination means that when we think about something deemed 'realistic' we think it is something you need to worry about.

For example, if I were to think about my car breaking down

on a journey leaving me stranded and missing appointments etc. that is not beyond reality and could be a source of worry. Then it becomes a debate as to how likely it is going to happen. If I said it was a very old car and has broken down four times in the last two weeks then it is more likely to happen and perhaps it might be worth thinking about mitigating that risk. However, if I said it is very new and has never broken down then you could say it is just my imagination and not to worry about it.

So using the definition of imagination being something that might not happen, or unrealistic, it becomes a debate as to whether something is likely to happen or not. The problem with this is our habitual over-thinking, our Outside-In Thought, makes things seem bigger than they are. It links our well-being with them so they are scarier and the fear of them is larger. The impact of them could be seen as compromising our well-being, happiness or security. So we worry about them happening more. We lose perspective.

We can quickly get caught in a debate in our head as to the likelihood of it happening and what we can do to prevent it from happening. It's not until the next day when our mind has settled and we have regained clarity we wonder what all the fuss was about.

I would like to suggest a different definition of imagination. If imagination was anything that is not in the present moment then it is clearer what is real and what isn't.

We spend a lot of our time worrying about things that haven't happened yet and we don't really know if they are going to happen. So, if anything that isn't in the present moment is imagination we can then see it for what it is, imagination, not reality. It may be plausible or realistic but any thought that is not in the present moment is not reality so it's imagination. Nothing can predict the future so it's imagination. And our human operating system is not designed for our imagination, it's designed for reality.

You may begin to notice as you do this you begin to see it with greater perspective. You become more grounded in your amazing range of resources in this moment and can look at the situation with greater insight, wisdom and clarity.

This does not mean not to think about the future, plan things, prepare for future events. Planning and preparation are good things to do. However, there is a different mindset with this kind of thinking about the future. When you purposefully think about the future, whether planning, visioning or preparing, you know you are looking at the future from the present moment. You are grounded in this moment and your resourcefulness knowing you are making an estimate about the future. You are looking at the future from an Inside-Out perspective. Knowing you are OK and your wisdom shows up in each moment when you need it.

When you get caught up in worry about the future you don't realise you are no longer in this moment. You are imagining yourself in a future reality and you think your Okness in some way is dependant on a particular outcome. You've gone Outside-In.

As humans, we are designed and equipped to deal with reality. This moment. The 'us' in our imaginary future is not the fully resourced us, so no wonder it feels scary.

Come back to now.

Come back to reality.

You've got it covered.

24

Fear of failure

M any of my clients have a fear of failure. Fear of not being successful in getting pregnant. Fear of not having everything they think a baby will give them. This can often be contentment, love or purpose. For me it was contentment. I didn't believe we would be as happy or fulfilled without children as with. I was scared of never being truly happy. Thus I was scared of not succeeding in having children.

This fear undermined all the good stuff I did to improve my fertility.

When we explore this fear of failing or not succeeding more it usually has been prevalent in the client's life for a long time. Not always about fertility but a fear of not succeeding. Perhaps growing up there was an expectation to achieve. I know with my Mum being a strict school-teacher who had a lot of anxious Thought she was scared me and my siblings wouldn't be OK unless we did 'well' at school. There was an expectation that we would work hard and do well, whatever 'well' meant in her eyes. In her eyes, it meant very well! Part of me unconsciously was scared I wouldn't be fully loved and accepted for who I was if I didn't achieve her standards.

I've never met anyone who doesn't have fear in their life in one form or another.

Fear isn't necessarily a bad thing. Fear isn't something we need to get rid of. Fear can be useful information. Are you in danger? Walking to close to a cliff edge can feel uneasy and fearful – that is giving you useful information that you may be putting yourself in danger. However chronic fear, a pretty common feeling of fear, isn't helpful and can undermine our well-being and your chances of getting pregnant.

What we want is a more healthy relationship with fear. It's about recognising it but not going for a ride with it.

Firstly, it's about recognising it's based on a presumption you are not OK unless you do/achieve something in this physical world. This is a misunderstanding of where your well-being comes from. We are born with it. It's inside us. It's innate and not dependant on anything. We may not feel OK a lot of the time, that's because we have lots of Outside-In Thought that tells us we are OK unless…

Secondly, it's being aware that Thought, even fearful Thought, is spontaneous and always based on reality. It's often stories in our head.

A fearful thought is like a taxi at a busy taxi stand. They come and they go. That's OK. They come, we can check the danger and then it can move on again. However often they arrive, we forget it's not real, it's a misuse of imagination, and get in and go for a ride with the fear.

The thing that makes us open the door of the taxi and go for a ride with the fear is falling for the illusions that it is real when there is no present danger. It is a psychological fear. Believing the feeling of fear is coming from what we think is going to happen. However, nothing can predict the future, not even your fearful thinking. And whatever happens, you are going to be OK as everything you need at any moment arrives in the moment. We are built for reality.

When we understand that our feelings know nothing about our circumstances or the future, we are feeling our thinking at the moment, nothing else, and we can begin to realise we don't need to go for a ride with it. We can notice it for what it is, a thought about the future.

When we understand we are OK, period, that who we are, our love-ability and OKness is not dependant on external achievements or any external yard-stick, we can change our relationship with fear. We can more easily see it for what it is. Habitual fearful Thought, not reality. We can let the cab go, knowing it's not something we have to pay attention to. Fresh Thought and perspective will be along any moment.

25

❖

The truth about affirmations

L ike us and many of my clients (when they first come to me) you are probably doing everything you can to ensure you maximise your chances of getting pregnant. One thing a lot of people think is key is positive thinking. Having a positive mindset surely is key. Hence affirmations can be popular.

My son had just walked to the top of a waterfall on a climb of 1,000 feet, aged three, wearing crocs! He was exhausted and extremely hungry. The thing was, the food and drink were a little back down the path with my wife (who was too scared to make the final vertical ascent). He was too tired to go another step but it was just too dangerous to even consider carrying him. 'I can't do it' he exclaimed bursting into tears from tiredness and hunger. I told him to say, 'I can do it, I can do it, I can do it,' out loud three times. When he did so his physiology changed and he immediately started the descent.

Affirmations can work. Most of the clients I see use them and you can see the effect, however, they are subconsciously using negative affirmations such as 'I'm not good enough' or 'I'm not going to ever be a Mum'. One of my common ones used to be 'I don't deserve good things'. I became aware of many of mine during in the midst of our fertility journey. These negative thoughts and beliefs create fear and tension in your mind and body which is not going to be helping you get pregnant.

Many people get this and the common way to try and be more positive and combat the habitual fearful and negative thinking is to use positive affirmations. It seems logical. Replace one set of thinking with something more useful. And the idea is if you do them enough they become the new subconscious, habitual thought patterns.

Hmm, good luck with that one!

The problem is two-fold. Fighting thought with thought generally does not work. Our habitual Outside-In thought processes think they are helping to survive in life. They genuinely think they are protecting your survival. It's the emotional brain seeking the answers for peace, love and security in the wrong place. Based on misunderstandings often from childhood. So replacing it with new thinking through repetition of phrases that part of you may not fully believe is unlikely to work.

Combatting thought with thought rarely works, which is why going upstream to understand the true nature of Thought helps us see through the Outside-In illusion it creates.

Another reason affirmations don't work is that they can be built upon fear. Fear of not being OK. Fearful Thought that believes you will not be OK unless you are successful in creating a specific external circumstance (e.g. better job, the baby). It believes you won't achieve this unless you have a more positive mindset. It can be like being on a knife-edge of 'OKness'.

Affirmations can be a bit like first aid and can help you in times of trouble but are not sustainable in creating a deeper sense of well-being and peace of mind.

What if you KNEW you were OK regardless of what Thought or feelings you were experiencing? What if you KNEW you would be OK whatever happens?

What if you didn't need any affirmations?

The only thing that stops us knowing we are OK is Thought telling us otherwise. It may be thought that has been there a long time, a belief about yourself, but it's still thought in this moment. Our tendency is to try and stop this negative thinking and move us to a more positive state of mind. We tend to think the negative thinking is bad.

What if this trying to be more positive is actually doing your more harm than good? Our mind has a self-correcting system. Left to its own devices it is always moving back to peace of mind, our innate well-being. The only thing that stops it is us trying to be OK. Is us not thinking we are OK if we don't feel OK.

If we recognise that 100% of your experience is thought that comes and goes, we don't have to be scared of any of our experiences, including our negative ones of fearful thinking. The more we see them for what they are, clouds of thought passing through, they know nothing about our circumstances or future, we can ALLOW them to be. We can fully allow our experience and it moves on. It's never our thinking or feeling that's the problem – it's whether we think it's a problem.

However, understanding the true nature of thought and connecting to your innate well-being that is always there, often masked by thought, can transform your experience in life far beyond the use of affirmations.

I believe allowing whatever experience to be, knowing where it's come from – Thought not 'reality' – is far more powerful than any affirmation. Acceptance of what you are feeling in any moment does not mean giving up. Far from it. It means allowing the noise & stories in your head and being in the present moment, knowing it knows nothing about your future. When we let go of trying to manage our thoughts we drop into a space below our thought, the default state of peace and well-being we were born with.

If you really want an affirmation, the one I recommend is 'I accept myself as I am today'.

In what way can you begin to accept yourself as you are today?

26

❖

Our innate well-being

I've talked a lot about the nature of Thought and where our experience comes from. I want to now turn our attention further to where our well-being comes from. On my own fertility journey I uncovered a sense of not being OK within myself. I thought I needed to 'prove' my value/worth to people, that they wouldn't love or like me for who I was. The same is true for many of my clients. This undercurrent of fear of not being OK or good enough is a source of stress and tension that is not going to be helping you get pregnant.

On my journey of exploration into the principles behind our human experience, I spent a lot of time understanding the nature of Thought and how Thought creates our experience. For the first time, I could begin to see how my experience was not coming from my circumstances. This was quite a revelation to me. However, I was somewhat still feeling anxious and fearful. I knew it was Thought but I didn't know how to stop it. At that point, I still thought there was something I had to do or change for me to feel different. I hadn't quite comprehended it is about not doing anything. About knowing I was OK whether I felt OK or not. One of the things preventing me from seeing this more clearly was an underlying belief that I was not OK.

I've mentioned before, I grew up with a mother who suffered from anxiety, was incredibly strict and had high expectations of me and my siblings. At a young age, I quickly learnt what I had to do to not be shouted at and thus to feel more loved and accepted. I was also brought up in an Anglo-Catholic church environment that talked of a God of unconditional love but all I could hear were the conditions between me and that love. I heard a lot about being a sinner and the need to repent. In my young mind from both home and church (and probably school) unconsciously I didn't believe I was OK for who I was.

One of the key principles of our human experience is the formless energy behind the life that enables life to hang together. The energy behind life that existed before time. It's the design behind life that enables a seed to become an apple tree, to bear fruit, and create more seeds. It's whatever God, the universe, mother nature, the energy behind life is for you. It's divine, loving, and creative. It's love in its purest form. We are made of that energy, we are part of that energy. It doesn't make anything that needs to prove itself.

I got that intellectually. I intellectually knew that God loved me unconditionally but didn't feel it. I knew as an adult my mum loved me unconditionally all my life. As a child, I often didn't feel it. I was desperate to feel that from her and from life. I wanted to grasp this unconditional love and acceptance and hold onto it like being enveloped in a hug of pure love and acceptance. Elsie Spittle has been sharing this psychology of the mind for over 30 years. She embodies love. She once talked about this energy behind life as receiving a hug. She said when she heard people talking a lot about Thought she could often see they needed to experience this energy behind life and she just wanted to give them a hug.

Because I thought I had to do something to be OK, I thought I had to do something in order to experience that feeling of unconditional acceptance.

It struck me like a bolt between the eyes when talking to some friends about the Inside-Out nature of our experience. He said when you look at a beautiful scene in nature, the scene is neutral, you are looking from a place of beauty. I had never considered this. I assumed I was looking at something beautiful that I was appreciating.

But if it really is an Inside-Out experience 100% of the time, then it is true. These are principles of our human experience which by the definition of a principle are consistent and predictable. It is the case 100% of the time.

Whatever you're looking at is neutral. The experience comes from within. So when you feel love and experience beauty it is coming from within you. It cannot come from anywhere else. And there's nothing you need to do to make that happen. It's within you whether you know it or not.

I used to listen to talks desperate to get a sense of that feeling of love and acceptance. It was like I was trying to grab a feather. Desperately listening for the words that would make the difference, that would unlock something within me. But it wasn't until I stopped trying, stopped listening to the words for the answer and listen to what was within me as the words washed over my experience I began to feel a feeling of acceptance and love within me.

The first time I really could sense it, it was a powerful feeling of self-compassion. Of knowing I was OK regardless of all the things I'd done that I wasn't proud of. Regardless of not being the person I thought I should be. Of knowing I was OK with who I was. It was like I could stop. Stop performing. Stop trying to live up to everyone's (and my unconscious) expectations.

So many of my clients have a similar experience. Part of them is trying to meet these unspoken expectations. Of trying to be

OK and prove to the world that they are just as worthy as everyone else on this planet. Fear of not being good enough. Of failing. Even failing to get pregnant.

What unconditional acceptance and love was your birthright? Because it is. It's not something you have to earn. It's who you are. You are a diamond. Perfect, pure and unique. We are imperfect humans because that's what being human is about. This is not about being perfect and being a Zen Buddhist master that is 100% in a state of inner peace. Not only is that impossible, it'd also be very boring!

This is about embracing our humanness, our personal weirdness but knowing we are OK regardless of that. Our souls are perfect. We are made of that energy behind life. We co-create our life with it.

Stop trying to be OK, to be acceptable, to be good enough. You are OK. More than OK. Do you know that?

27

❖

Steering the roller-coaster of life

Fertility is often referred to as an emotional roller-coaster. The ups of hope and possibility can quickly crash down to devastation, grief and hopelessness. When we finally had our positive pregnancy test I didn't want to believe it as we'd had false hopes in the past only for them to be snatched away. I didn't want to get my hopes up because I couldn't take more bad news.

But life is also a roller-coaster. The ups and downs and twists and turns of everyday life may not be as steep and high as an emotional fertility roller-coaster, but life is still unpredictable and things happen that are not of our choosing.

When we feel the need to try and control circumstances and outcomes in order to know we are going to be OK or create the things we think we need to be happy, it can be like trying to steer a roller-coaster. It can get rather uncomfortable.

Firstly it is futile because nothing can predict the future, not even your thinking, no matter how hard you fret over it. Trying to control outcomes and worrying about future events only brings stress, anxiety and unhappiness.

The future is an incomplete equation by its nature. I've spent much of my life trying to resolve it. Trying to make sure I am going to be OK, or ensure I create the circumstances I need to be

OK. Many secondary fertility clients think that their child needs a sibling otherwise it won't be as happy or will be lonely in life. How do they know that if they did have siblings that they would get on? I know plenty of adults who rarely speak to their siblings or who actively don't like each other. Like most of my clients, I genuinely believed we wouldn't be as happy without our own children as with. Prior to that, I thought I needed a good career to be happy and secure in life or needed to find a partner to be happy.

Don't get me wrong, there is nothing wrong with any of those things, but it's the future imagination that our life will be better because of it. That leads to the fear of it not happening and a lot of future thinking trying to ensure the tracks of life are going in the direction you think you need. It stops you being open to other possibilities. We create blinkers that stop us seeing opportunities in the moment that may not be the path we expected but may take us to either a better place or the place we desired via a different route.

Imagine looking forward to going for a Chinese meal on a Friday night. All week you are looking forward to it. You know the restaurant well and you know exactly what you are going to order. What happens when the time comes and you go into town and see some old friends. You get talking and they ask you to join them for an Italian. What do you do? Say no, and stick to your original plan and not be open to the possibility of something different? Perhaps. You could go with them. They could come with you. You could arrange to meet at another time. What happens if you get to your Chinese restaurant and when you order the crispy duck you've been expecting all week they say it's not on the menu that night? How does that feel having been expecting it all week?

There is nothing wrong with wanting something and looking

forward to it. Having a meal may be a frivolous example. With bigger things in life, we can tend to take it further beyond a desire, to think we need it. That there isn't really any other option because nothing else would satisfy you. What if that were not true?

Another aspect of steering the roller-coaster is trying to avoid the lows in life. Trying to keep us on the straight and level. To avoid the emotional bits. We are addicted to feeling comfortable because we think we are OK if we feel OK.

The more we know where our well-being comes from and where our human experience comes from we no-longer have to be scared of any experience in life. We can relax on the roller-coaster ride of life knowing whatever happens we will be OK.

We can have what we judge to be an unpleasant experience and still know we are OK. It can be a little weird being aware of that for the first time. Feeling sad, angry, or whatever it may be, but underneath the feeling still knowing we are OK. It means we can fully allow it and fresh perspectives come through more quickly than we imagine.

I love this roller-coaster metaphor for life from Michael Neill's book Super Coach[1]:

Imagine that you are riding on a giant barge, floating gently down a beautiful river. In the very centre of the barge is a giant roller coaster, and your seat for the journey is in the front car. As the river carries the barge downstream, the roller coaster goes up and down, pausing every now and again before climbing its way to the next peak or plunging its way down into the valleys. At times it spins wildly, completely disorienting you; at other times you find yourself resting in the pause before the next ride.

Now imagine that your whole life, you had ridden the coaster with your eyes closed, believing that the roller coaster was the world and the river only a myth. What would happen the first time you opened your eyes and kept them open for every moment of the ride?

At first, you might be a bit disoriented and even frightened as you watched yourself and others go up and down and round and around at occasionally dizzying speeds. The first time you crested the heights of the coaster and saw the river clearly in all its glory, you would be so taken by the view that you would never want it to end. And when your revelation was followed by a plunge to the bottom of your world it might seem like all was lost.

But over time, you would begin to relax into the ride, spending less and less time trying to manage the ups and downs and more and more time enjoying the views along the way. You'd take comfort in the fact that no matter what was going on with the roller coaster, the river was always effortlessly supporting the barge along its journey. And you might even begin to enjoy pondering the mysteries of where the river came from, how you came to be on it, and where it might be taking you…

28

❖

Owner v victim

I want to explore what's behind a word that I hear clients use quite often. The word is 'should'. We all use it from time to time but often don't understand the negative impact of the mindset behind it. What are you doing as part of your journey to getting pregnant because you think you 'should'. What about life as a whole? What are you doing because you think you 'should'? No-one likes being told what to do even if it is ourselves doing the telling!

At any point in time, we are either operating as a creator or victim of our life. We can either feel empowered, resilient and ready to face whatever life brings up or we can feel powerless, resigned to our experience of circumstances believing it can't be any different.

I can look back and see how much I was a victim in life. I wasn't aware of it at the time. It wasn't until I accepted I wasn't happy in life. I then could see with more clarity that one of the reasons I wasn't happy was I was angry that 'life' hadn't returned its part of the bargain. I had worked hard, been a 'good boy' done everything I thought I should. I wasn't fair that others seemed to get what they wanted in life, as well as happiness, far more easily than me. I believed for some reason life was harder for me. And it wasn't fair. I was angry. I felt like a victim. But it left me feeling powerless, with nowhere to go – that 'life' had all the power. That's not a comfortable or enjoyable place to be.

Nor is it how we are designed to be.

I think there are three approaches to life (this is a model, not truth). One is striving for what you think you need to be happy. To do everything you can to make it happen. This is usually fuelled by fear of it not happening. We think that it's empowering as we feel in control, but actually it puts all the power into the physical world. The power to make us happy. That our happiness is dependant on the external event coming to fruition. And if it doesn't for whatever reason we are left feeling angry and resentful. That we've done our part and 'life' is not doing theirs.

Another approach that can be popular is the law of attraction. To think what you want into your life and this metaphysical abundant energy behind life will bless you with it. The problem with this is that; a) it is often fuelled by fear of not obtaining those things you think you need to be happy so; b) it again puts all the power outside of us to the metaphysical energy behind life.

However, I think there is a third way. I do believe in a divine, loving and abundant metaphysical energy behind life. However, I also believe we are made of it and part of it. And as we are part of it we co-create our life with it. That we have all the resources we need to thrive in this world. This is empowering. Look at toddlers, they don't rely on anything external to create amazing experiences of learning to walk and talk, to explore this wonderful world from a place of wonder.

I love Life Coach Steve Chandler's differentiation between being an owner and a victim. It matches the differentiation of seeing our human experience being Inside-Out v Outside-in.

Owners take ownership of their response to a situation. We cannot choose the circumstances. But the more we understand that nothing makes us feel anything, and our experience is coming from Thought, we tend to have a wider range of resource to choose a response that empowers us. A victim thinks their experience is coming from the circumstances. It's being done 'to them'.

Owners see life as an energy of potential. A source of possibility to be used. A victim sees life as using them. That life is unfair, a burden. Steve tells a story of how a woman came to see him at the end of the talk he had given. She told him how she was teaching her children life is unfair. How she constantly reminded them of that. When she saw them being happy going off the school she would remind them life is unfair. When they were looking peaceful and going to sleep she would remind them that life isn't fair. Steve was obviously quite taken aback by this but asked what her question was. She asked 'why are my children so depressed all the time'. 'Oh I don't know?!' he says with his dry sense of humour!

Victims use the word 'should'. Nothing is more disempowering than the word 'should'. It doesn't motivate you to get on and do whatever it is. No-one likes being told what to do, even if it is ourselves doing the telling! However, it's usually other people's thoughts and beliefs we've picked up over the years and are behind our use of the word. It's not coming from our soul. It's Outside-In Thought. Our soul is a place of creativity and empowerment. An owner makes a choice of doing something even if it is something part of them doesn't want to do. If they think it's aligned to their soul, even though they know they are not necessarily going to enjoy it, they don't say they 'should' do it. They make a choice of doing it. They are owning the choice instead of having the experience of life making them do it.

An owner will see a situation and ask how they can use it. Even if it's a situation not of their choosing or a problem. They take a step back and see it from a different perspective, allow clarity to come and see what they can create from it. Whether it be better relationships, tighter agreements or other learning. They find the hidden gem in the situation that is almost always there. Victims ask why it's happening to them and resent the experience.

Owners will ask 'what can I do' about a situation. A victim will feel powerless. When you feel powerless you lose focus, creativity, and perspective. All the things required to create something and achieve the things you want in life.

An owner doesn't need a reason to be happy. They see it works Inside-Out. How happiness is an inside job. Happiness is what you bring to things not what you get from them. Victims need people, places, or situations to make them happy. They think it works Outside-In.

Owners come from a place of being. They ask themselves who do I need to be to make this happen. They can see our sense of self is limited to Thought in this moment. Thought changes moment to moment. Therefore who we are is flexible. There is no fixed sense of self. Victims say it's just the way they are and can't see any possibility of change.

At any point in time ask yourself are you being an owner of a victim?

29

❖

Expectations

"We must let go of the life we have planned, so as to accept the one that is waiting for us." Joseph Campbell

I want to explore how we can have expectations and how they can impact our sense of happiness and well-being and be a source of distress, frustration and disappointment.

Let's look at an example. A friend told me they had met someone who had fallen in love with their wife 14 years before they actually got together. They'd been friends for a long time. He had been admiring her. In fact, he had fallen in love with her and never really believed or thought that she would have any affection back. This went on for 14 years.

Finally, when they did get together she invited him back to her place. They were talking and she said, "Would you like to stay over?" And he said, "No, Because I don't think I could ever live up to how I have imagined over the last 14 years".

It's interesting how in our expectations, we imagine how something's going to be. It's like a movie playing out in the back of our mind. We forget it's not real. Especially if we play it out often, it does become how we think things should be and can't imagine it being any different. It becomes the benchmark and anything less is not going to be good.

Society can create expectations about how life should be. The Disney fairy tale story, princess meets prince charming. They have children and they all live happily ever after. For me, my parents had expectations of me. Expectations that I'll be successful, get the good grades, be the achiever.

Over times these expectations become our expectations. They become the filter we look at our life through. We then worry that if our life is not meeting these expectations, that we're not going to reach the benchmark of what we think we need to be fully content or happy.

Expectations can be present in all areas of our lives and they can be particularly prevalent in relationships.

Expectations often lead to disillusionment or disappointment and prevent us from having more gratitude and appreciation of life. Let me explain why.

When expectations are present, if they are met, then we often don't feel anything particular. We are neutral about it because we expected that thing to happen. Nothing to get excited about as it's what we expected.

If expectations are exceeded we might have a good feeling about it. However when they are not met that often leads to feelings such as disillusionment, disappointment, or frustration.

So expectations prevent us from having an appreciation of situations, people, ourselves and life.

Imagine a couple move in together and every morning the man gets up to make a cup of tea for them to enjoy in bed before they start their day. His partner really appreciates this, especially on the cold dark mornings. She has appreciation and gratitude. However, if after a while it becomes an expectation, she will lose her appreciation and gratitude because it's what she expected to happen. Once it's an expectation and it doesn't happen it can lead to disappointment or even frustration.

Expectations can dramatically reduce our levels of happiness and appreciation of life and increase our levels of dissatisfaction or annoyance.

Expectations are unspoken agreements. These can be toxic in any situation but particularly relationships (whether romantic, friends or work).

If a boss expects certain standards of behaviour or targets, the staff may think that those expectations are unreasonable. Maybe they believe they're under-resourced to achieve them. No-one likes to have expectations put on them and it can create a resentment in the relationship. In a work situation if staff are involved in creating standards and targets they are far more committed to making them happen.

Sometimes, if you talk to a boss about their expectations they would say, "The staff knew what I was expecting". It's still not an agreement. They're putting something on to someone without actually agreeing to it.

What's interesting also is that expectations put the responsibility on to the other person. So if a boss has expectations that their staff delivers a report by a certain date without having a conversation and clear agreement it puts all the responsibility onto the other person. It's not a two-way agreement. It's a one-way flow.

I had an expectation that getting married would make me happy. This was an unconscious belief. I wasn't fulfilled or happy but wasn't consciously aware of that. I wasn't aware I was looking for people and situations to change that, to make me happy.

Because I went into the relationship with unrealistic expectations as the relationship matured past the loved-up honeymoon period I was back to being discontent. So I began looking for the next thing that would make us happy (I thought if 'we' were happy I would be happy, aka if my wife is happy I would be happy).

Having a baby will make us happy! I am positive that this expectation contributed to my infertility. It was locking me into a victim Outside-In mentality. Which leads to dis-ease which creates tension and stress in our body. There is a school of thought that a lot of disease comes from dis-ease in the mind affecting the body.

The truth is I wasn't happy even before I got married, even though I had everything society says you need to be happy (the good career, health, hobbies, friends, etc.). That's why I was looking for something else to make me happy. But that's the Outside-In approach to living life, the 'I'll be happy when…' keeps you on a merry-go-round looking for the next thing because it's looking in the wrong place for contentment.

As well as expectations of other people, we can have expectations of ourselves. Expectations of the type of person we should be or the level of success we think we should be creating or where we should be in life by now. Again, these expectations can lead to disillusionment and frustration towards ourselves and life.

Expectations take us away from the present moment and the reality of the situation. We go into the la-la land of how life 'should' be in our heads. Expectations are fighting reality. Fighting reality never leads to a good result!

When we let go of expectations we can come back to be present to what is. To accept reality. To re-connect to our innate well-being in this moment. To see things with greater perspective, resourcefulness, as a creator rather than a victim.

What expectations do you have on yourself?

What expectations do you have on others?

What expectations do you have for life?

How would you be if you could begin to let those go and be more present and alive to this moment?

30

❖

Being in the here & now

I am a keen runner. My running has taught me a lot about being in the moment. I used to run with my music on, head down and powering through the miles and striving to complete the distance. I would constantly be aware of how far I needed to go, what hills were coming up and ensuring I would have enough energy to achieve my goal.

When I started running barefoot it enabled me to be more fully present to my experience. Being able to feel the ground, how my body was interacting with it, enabled me to be more present to that moment. I was more aware of my body and our body is always in the present moment. I quickly stopped running with music and enjoyed being more aware of my surroundings, my body and my experience. Running became like a meditation for me.

What surprised me was how much more I enjoyed my running but also how my running improved as a result. One factor is because the barefoot running style is more efficient for your body. However, a huge factor was not being limited by my thinking. I thought the analysis of my run in my head was helping me pace myself or push myself to achieve greater goals. But I found with a calmer mind and being more present to my body I achieved more with greater ease. Whilst I had set a conscious intent of how far I wanted to run, I held it lightly as I was more present to what I was experiencing at the moment. It was like my body knew what I wanted to achieve and all I needed to do was listen to it whilst being present and it enabled me to achieve my distances with greater ease.

My body was far more able than I thought it was. On a training run, I had to complete six hill sprints of 90 seconds each. In my head when I set out before my warm up, I thought I only had to do four. My watch was clearly telling me six. I thought there was no way I could do six and thought perhaps I'll be able to do four and that will be enough. Then I had an insight. I would start all six whether I finished them or not. To my amazement, I did all six and the last two were the best! They felt the most relaxed and the most effortless.

In all of life, we can achieve things far greater than we ever think when we ignore our habitual Outside-In thinking, which includes our limiting thoughts and beliefs.

When we hold our goals lightly, whilst being present to the moment, the creative energy between these two moves us forward in a state of flow.

Outside-In Thought is always about the past and the future. It genuinely thinks it's there to help. It wants us to be happy, safe and fulfilled. However because it is looking in the wrong place for those things, looking in this world of form (of circumstances, situations and people) it never achieves it. So we stay in our heads going round and round trying to achieve what we want. Tying ourselves into bigger and bigger knots.

Your mind can time travel but your body can't. Come back to the here and now, back to where your body and soul are.

Utilising the 3-5 breathing technique from chapter 15 is a great way of doing just that.

When I find at times I am overwhelmed by thinking I often imagine a glitter ball or snow globe in my head, each bit of glitter representing an Outside-In Thought, settling without needing me to do anything because I don't need resolving Thought. It is a self-correcting system. Fresh perspectives and Thought come in automatically when we stop interfering with the system, stop trying to think our way back to peace of mind. Visualising it settling in my head helps me come back to the present moment and be more aware of my body and my true sense of self.

When I do that my mind begins to settle and I regain clarity on circumstances and re-connect to my innate well-being that is within us all the time.

Amazing things can happen when you begin to be present and connect to your body. You can hear your body, it can help guide you to what's best for you on your journey to getting pregnant. As we'll dive in to later, it's also where you can guide it to do amazing things too.

Have fun coming back to the here and now and being more aware of your body. Put your hand on your womb, breathe in to that space. What does it want to say to you? I know that sounds a bit crazy, but give it a go! Your body has wisdom that surpasses our thinking.

31

❖

You are not your thinking

There's an old Sufi joke. It goes like this. There was once a drunk man scrabbling under a lamppost in the middle of the night. A policeman comes along and asks what he's doing. The drunk man looks up and tells him that he's lost his keys. The policeman says he will help look and asks him where he dropped them. The drunk man points to the other side of the road and says 'over there'. Confused, the policeman asks 'So why are you looking here?'. The man replies 'Because the light is better over here!'

Our Outside-In Thought does the same thing.

It looks for emotional well-being, peace of mind and happiness in the wrong place. It looks for meaning and our sense of self in the wrong place.

It looks in the obvious place, what we can see in our physical world. In the world of form. When we look in this direction we are looking downstream of the effects of Thought and not upstream towards our true sense of self, capabilities and resources.

Outside-In Thought genuinely believes that our emotional well-being is dependent on things outside of us. For example, 'I'm OK if…' or 'I'm OK when…' This creates a very busy mind trying to manage all the possibilities of what may or may not happen in order to create the outcome your thinking thinks you need.

This is looking downstream from our true sense of self and looking at who we think we are rather than who we really are. As a result, we feel insecure and look for what we think we need to be OK. Again we look in the obvious place, where what we can see, the world of form for OKness. However, everything we need in this moment is within us already. We were born with it. And what we need for every future moment will again be there within us when we need it. That's how the human operating system works.

All the greatest spiritual teachings over the millennia say the same thing, 'look within'. We often don't do this because we don't like what we see, but that is who we think we are, not who we really are.

It can be easier to see when other people are caught in their Outside-In thinking which is not true, but often we don't see when we are doing the same thing. It's too convincing and too scary to trust that it can't be real.

Growing up I felt I couldn't relax. If I let go and went with the flow of what I wanted to do something bad usually happened. I ended up getting shouted at. In the back of my mind, I can habitually think that is how life is. It's not safe to relax and be, you have to be on high alert and think things through to prevent bad things from happening. It's as if I'm not OK unless I make sure things are in place to make sure I'm OK.

This is Outside-In. This is what many of us learn from life growing up whether subtly or overtly. But it's not true. It's not who we are or how life works. When was the last time you saw a baby and thought they weren't OK? Weren't a complete and perfect soul in that moment?

We are born as a diamond, perfect and unique. Then things happen in life. Whether through upbringing, school system, kids in the playground, we start to think our OKness is dependant on things on the outside. Perhaps on what parents, teachers or friends think of us. Perhaps keeping our parents together and them not arguing. It is like horse manure gets thrown at the diamond. And sometimes it sticks.

Before we know it, all we see is a pile of horse manure. And we don't like what we see. We are worried about what people might think of us. We work really hard to polish the pile of horse manure, to give it a shine, giving an impression that we are OK. Or we mask up and project an image of being OK, like putting a layer of nail polish around the pile of horse manure.

However, all along we have forgotten we are actually the diamond.

We think we are the pile of manure. That we are not 100% acceptable as we are. That people won't love and likes us for who we are. Worrying about what people might think of us. The manure is habitual Outside-In Thought telling us our sense of being OK is dependant on something outside of us.

It started in all innocence. When we are young all we want is unconditional positive regard from our caregivers and others around us. If for any reason we don't get that we think what we need to think to get that. My being a 'good boy' meant that I felt more loved and was shouted at less than perhaps otherwise. However, these Thought habits continue out of habit when we grow up and no longer need them. They become what creates our habitual perception of life and ourselves.

When we begin to see this illusion we can stop fighting it. We can realise it's not who we are. It's not the way life is. When we allow it, for what it is, Thought, it settles automatically. When we see it as our habitual flavour of Thought we don't need to do anything about it. We automatically begin to connect with our true self, the diamond, the beautiful, complete person that came into this world as a baby.

The true self you get glimpses of when you have a quieter mind. The true self that has insight, inspiration and connection to people and nature around you. Connected to life. Connected to the present moment.

That's who you really are. Do you know that?

Chasing your thinking brings stress and anxiety. Connecting back to your true self allows your mind and body to become back in balance. Back in to flow. Back in to the healthiest state it can be for you to get pregnant.

32

❖

Our true identity

As well as emotional distress being a familiar experience, infertility can also question or challenge our sense of identity as a woman or man. When we can't do what seems to be a very natural biological function, some believing reproduction is the core purpose of our existence, we can begin to question our sense of womanhood or manhood. Part of me felt less of a man because I couldn't have children. Something that felt to be at the biological core of what it means to be a man. I know my wife felt the same about her infertility.

It begs the question as to where we get our sense of identity from. It wasn't until I left my career of 17 years working for a large well-known company I realised how much my identity was tied up with my job. I was proud of who I worked for and I thought my job title made me a more interesting person. That people would be more interested in me because of what I did rather than who I am as a person. Ultimately, I was more proud of what I did than who I was. This meant I was more attached to the identity of the job title rather than any other sense of who I was.

So what is our identity? Who are we? If the doorbell went and my son called out to say a tax inspector was at the door for me, then one kind of Russell will probably show up at the door. If my son called out to say Julia Roberts was at the door for me, I imagine a very different Russell to show up at the door!

I think trying to answer the question 'Who are you?' points us in the wrong direction. It points us to a lot of ego thought. Outside-In thinking about who we think we are in this physical world, in this world of form. I think we get more answers and understanding looking further upstream, by asking the question 'What are you?'. It may seem an odd question to consider but I think it points us upstream from ego Thought, to a place that existed before our sense identity, before who we think we are in this physical world.

I see us as being spiritual beings having a physical experience. Our soul is formless and the observer of our the human experience. For example, when you are debating with yourself in your head about a decision you need to make you can see two sides of the argument. Two 'yous' each giving their case. Which one is the real you? Which one should you listen to? The real you is neither of them. The real you is the observer of the debate. Neither is your true self. Both are Thought. You are the observer of all Thought and the corresponding experience it creates.

I liken us to an iceberg. If the formless loving creative energy behind life was the ocean, we are made of water. An iceberg. A very small percentage of us is above the water, in this world of form having a human experience. Often that's all we think we are. Seeking to find understanding and well-being in this world of form. But we are also everything below the water. Our soul is this formless energy made of the divine loving energy behind life. That's who we really are. We are the observer of the human experience.

When we feel at peace and connected in the moment we feel connected to our true sense of self, the space below Thought. We feel connected to the other people in the moment (if they too are calm and grounded to the moment) and we feel connected to the moment itself. What connects us to others and even nature in the moment is the energy that ties everything together. We are all made of it, part of it. When our sense of self in this moment melts in to the oneness of life we feel a sense of peace and clarity regardless of circumstances. We have less contaminated Outside-In Thought in the moment and are more present and connected to our true self, a feeling within that knows we are OK because it's not dependant on anything.

When we not aware of everything below the water, the source of our innate well-being, our grounding, we become like something floating on the water being tossed around by the waves of life. The more we become aware of our true sense of self, our soul that is the formless energy behind life, we feel more grounded. We know we are OK whether we feel OK or not. Knowing we are OK whatever happens.

This brings us to a place of peace. A place of peace without giving up. This is the place where the magic can happen!

33

❖

The answer's in the question

I think the role of a coach is to upgrade the quality of questions the client is asking themselves.

We often get in the habit of telling ourselves things, listening to our thinking (whether positive or negative) rather than asking ourselves questions. Statements are finite. Questions open up possibilities.

Recently I was really struggling with a run. I didn't have the energy in me. I had an insight that I was significantly upping my running training but I wasn't supporting this with my nutrition. I wasn't giving my body the right fuel.

Instead of telling myself I needed to lay off sugar and other unhelpful foods and to fuel myself with more nutrients, I asked myself the question, 'What do I need to do to allow myself to eat more healthily?'

The answer actually surprised me. It wasn't the 'stop eating sugar' or 'eat more carbs before a run' that I was expecting. The answer that came from within me was 'love yourself'. I know from that place I would naturally look after myself through my eating with more compassion and motivation than telling myself what I 'had' to do.

I remember when exploring my relationship with money I read the book, *Rich Dad Poor Dad* by Robert Kiyosaki. The book is about what the author learnt about money from his own dad and his best friend's dad. His father worked as a teacher and although the family were quite middle-class by most standards his father often said they couldn't afford things. By contrast, his best friend's dad, who at the time had less money than his real Dad, would ask himself the question 'how can we afford that?' His best friend's Dad went on to be very wealthy owning a string of businesses.

Questions open our minds to new possibilities.

For me, exploring questions rather than telling myself statements or judgements, I am always surprised how answers seem to come from within without trying. From our still soft voice of intuition. It's ever-present. It's always kind. Questions can open up space in our mind to allow the answer to float to the surface. From a place of love and inspiration that is more motivating than telling ourselves the things we need or should do.

We are brought up almost not to ask questions. To do what we are told and fall into line.

One way of helping yourself get more into a questioning mindset is to practice writing 10 questions a day. You don't even need to answer them, just get into the practice of asking yourself questions that expand your consciousness.

It is as simple as me asking myself 'what do I need to do to eat more healthily?' There is no right or wrong to this; follow your intuition.

To get you going here are some examples that may inspire you.

- What does loving myself today look like?
- What does it feel like to be open and willing to receive with ease?

- What questions do I need to ask to up-level my relationships with my partner, my health, happiness?
- What does it feel like to be ME?

So what question could you ask yourself that may open you up to a new possibilities for you on your fertility journey?

34

❖

Finding your intuition

"The solutions to outwardly complex problems created by misguided thoughts will not arise from complicated analytical theory, but will emerge as an insight, wrapped in a blanket of simplicity." Sydney Banks

This is one of my favourite quotes. I am a recovering 'thinkaholic'. Whether it was resolving a problem or re-designing a cornflake, I thought thinking was the way to solve all of my and life's problems! Surely a problem won't go away until you've thought of the solution? Let's explore that concept.

When do you have the best ideas? The best solutions to problems? When I ask people this question the answer is usually something like 'in the shower', 'driving' or 'walking the dog'. This is because at these times we are not consciously thinking about the problem. We have a quieter mind and space for new ideas, creativity and insights.

This is our intuition, our instinct, I call it our wisdom because it includes our knowledge, intellect and experience. We don't make whimsical decisions when we trust our instinct, we make wise ones. When was the last time you trusted your instinct and it let you down? We usually regret not listening to it. We get an idea of instinct about something but then our habitual outside-in thinking over-rides it and tells us all the reasons not to trust it.

We have two guidance mechanisms we experience. One is

Outside-In Thought founded on 'I'll be OK when/if…' and the other is Inside-Out Thought that knows our innate well-being, our true self and that whatever happens, we'll be OK. This gives mental space for possibilities, new ideas and fresh thinking. It allows us to access our amazing innate capabilities such as clarity, perspective, insight, creativity, direction. All this allows decisions to become easier and know the decision is aligned with our soul and not our fearful Outside-In Thought.

So do we differentiate between Outside-In Thought and our Inside-Out Thought that is grounded in intuition & wisdom? For me, there is a different energy between the two. Intuition is grounded in the here and now and comes with more of a sense of peace. Our Outside-In Thought is often grounded in fear.

Biological cells are in one of two states. Growth or protection[1]. When in growth they are multiplying. If they sense a threat in their environment the cells go into protection mode. They stop growing until the threat has passed. Given that we are a bunch of biological cells, we operate in much the same way psychologically.

Any decision can be approached from a perspective of growth or protection. Growth is understandably preferable. Humans naturally want to grow and develop. This leads us to live more of the life we want. We are not built to be stagnant. Children learn and grow intrinsically. Play is learning. They are learning new things about themselves and the world all the time. Toddlers learn to walk and talk without being in any toddler development school. Growth is intrinsic. Sometimes we need to be in a state of protection, survival mode but obviously overall a state of growth is preferable to a state of protection.

However, growth can feel scary. It can mean coming out of our comfort zone or leaning into our edge of fear. For example, it may be calling us to have a challenging conversation with a friend or deal with a difficult situation at work. It doesn't feel good but it feels right, in order to honour yourself and others. The thing is, outside our comfort zone is where the magic of life lives. It's where we step out of our fears and into our true self and can often feel more alive to life when we realise the fear that held us back was an illusion.

Protection is fuelled by fear. It wants to keep us in a place that feels safe and comfortable. To avoid fear and being uncomfortable. This keeps us in a prison of fear. Its intent is to avoid feeling uncomfortable. However, what feels comfortable in the short term feels uncomfortable in the long term as we are not aligned with our soul. For example, if someone wants to get fit, they know it's going to be good for them on every level, but it feels really uncomfortable to get out bed early to get to the gym before work. However, over time the short-term comfort they get from staying in bed feels uncomfortable because they know they are not honouring their soul's true desire.

So how do we hear our intuition? Firstly, it's being aware of the energy of our thoughts. Does it feel like growth or protection? What feels life-giving? Being more aware of the nature of our inner wisdom, intuition, can help you identify whether that is what you are tuned into or not.

Our intuition often comes in moments of quiet, it's an inner knowing that is often not backed up by logical argument, it is what feels right for us. The Outside-In Thought that contaminates our connection to our true self is fearful of you not being OK. As a result, it over thinks decisions bringing all the evidence from the past and its imaginary future as to why you should listen to it. It's very believable. But it's not reality. It's looking at things through fear-based goggles.

Our instinct factors into our past experiences and expertise but makes a decision-based in the here and now and knowing that whatever happens, you'll be OK. That allows you to grow and give birth to the life you want even if it means stretching your comfort zone.

Those days when you feel like you are on fire, at work getting things done, at the top of your game and it feels effortless. A state of flow. You are making decisions intuitively. That intuition includes your knowledge, intellect, life experience. You don't make whimsical decisions when you trust your instinct, it's your wisdom.

I love Michael Neill's description of the characteristics of wisdom in his book *Supercoach*[2]:

- Wisdom is ever present and always kind.
- Wisdom is sometimes soft but always clear.
- Wisdom comes most often in the midst of inner quiet.
- Wisdom feels right, even if it doesn't always feel good.
- Wisdom often comes disguised as 'common sense' but in reality is extremely uncommon in usage.

What does your inner wisdom say about your fertility journey? Is there anything it wants you to stop doing/do less of? Is there anything it wants you to start/do more of? What does it want to say to you? What do you sense as your truth in moments of quiet?

Enjoy exploring your inner wisdom!

---

1. Lipton, B. *Biology of Belief.* US: Hay House Inc; 2005; p149.

2. Neill, M. *Supercoach.* US: Hay House Inc; 2009, p102.

Part 3

Your Thinking & Your Body

35

❖

Tuning in to your body

How connected to your body do you feel?

I can be so in my head that I am often not aware of my body. I am sometimes unaware that I am sitting in an awkward position. I once worked on my laptop on a train for five hours (writing this book!), blissfully unaware how the position was damaging my neck and shoulder. That was until I woke up the next morning! It took me some time and lots of stretching to recover from that.

It can be surprising the number of clients that take a huge sigh and relax in to the moment when I bring their attention to their body. The shoulders drop and they land back into their body and the moment.

When we get caught in our thinking, our heads disconnect from our body. Our body is in the here and now, but our thinking is all about future stuff or past stuff; it takes us away from the here and now.

What's ironic is we are in our heads trying to work out what's best for our body but in doing so are disconnecting from the one thing that can help us with the answer. Our body wisdom.

Your body is the best doctor, nutritionist and life coach you will ever need. When you tune into your body you also tune into your inner wisdom.

For example, have you ever eaten something you regret? Either you weren't really hungry or it wasn't food that nourished you? Our body knows exactly when we are hungry or not. It also naturally craves nutrients, not sugar & chemical laden foods. When we are truly connected to our body in this moment we have innate satisfaction, we don't crave an external satisfaction kick or something to numb the dissatisfaction.

We overeat or eat things we regret when we are led by our Outside-In Thought and corresponding emotions. We are only ever living in the experience of Thought in this moment, which includes cravings. Outside-In Thought tells us we will feel better for eating the biscuit, but do we?! No, because it's looking in the wrong place for psychological well-being.

Getting out of our head and tuning into our bodies is a great way of re-connecting to your inner self. Your wisdom and intuition.

Your inner self is the best guide to life.

Your inner self is a place of love for yourself and others. A place of peace and security and wisdom. It will let you know what is best for you on your fertility journey. Instinct is your best guidance mechanism to life. It's not contaminated by fear of not getting pregnant. It is grounded in this moment and has clarity and perspective.

So how can you re-connect to your body/inner-self?

- You can use the 3-5 breathing exercise from chapter 15 as a way of tuning out of thinking and into your body. It can be a form of meditation.
- If you meditate, meditate on your body.
- Yoga is a great way of re-connecting to your body.
- I discovered Qigong and love it as a way of connecting to my body and getting my energy flowing within.
- Exercise is a great way of re-connecting to your body. Although be aware strenuous exercise can negatively impact

your fertility, which is why so many female athletes struggle with infertility.

- This may sound crazy but you may be surprised at the insights you get from it- talk to your body. Put your hand on your womb, breathe into it. Calm your mind and ask it what it needs or wants.

Re-connecting to my body has been one of the greatest joys of our fertility journey (of course, as well as having our son!). Each time I get an insight and shed another load of habitual Outside-In Thought I feel even more connected to my body. Over the years my diet and lifestyle have changed dramatically (for the better) and it's felt effortless as it's been me connecting to what my body instinctively wants.

When you connect to your body you are bringing your mind and body back into alignment. That's also a place where magic can happen, as we'll explore over the next few chapters.

36

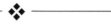

Mind and body – one system

Why is it when we have a nightmare we wake up with a racing heart and even perhaps in a cold sweat, when it was all in our mind?

Your mind and body are one system. Every part of your body is connected to your brain through nerves. When you are sad or happy and cry, your thoughts and feelings result in your body producing tears. Or an embarrassing thought can turn your face red.

Equally, what happens to the body registers in the brain, but the brain can influence exactly how it registers and to what degree. You may have noticed how a pain is reduced or goes away when you are distracted by something. The nerves are still connected but the mind is focussed on and registering something else.

I first learnt about the power of the mind when at the age of 16 I developed stage fright as a violinist (a shaking bow does not lead to a beautiful sound!). My violin teacher taught me some mind techniques that helped me let go of my nerves by stopping me focussing on my negative feelings and expecting my hand-shake to start imminently so that instead I could relax into my performance.

At the time I didn't really grasp the power of the principles of the mind behind the techniques and how they could have a far-reaching impact on all areas of my life. I do now.

I've even noticed recently when I am running, if my mind wanders and starts thinking about a challenging situation in life that I feel stuck in, I stop running. It's like mind overwhelm gets translated as physical overwhelm. It feels like I can't continue physically particularly if this happens towards the end of a run. However, it's not physical. It can happen in the middle of a regular route. It is my mind affecting my body. When I snap out of the trance and come back to the present moment I can continue on my way.

There are many examples of scientific research demonstrating the mind-body connection and the power of it.

Harvard psychologist Professor Ellen Langer has spent her entire career investigating the power of our mind. "Everybody knows in some way that our minds affect our physical being, but I don't think people are aware of just how profound the effect actually is," she says.

Prof. Langer's research started over 30 years ago in 1979 when she carried out a ground-breaking experiment. She wanted to know whether recreating a state of mind from 20 years earlier would make any changes in the bodies of participants, and indeed, the results showed profound and positive differences that were truly amazing.

Prof. Langer recruited a group of elderly men all in their late 70s or 80s for a "week of reminiscence". Surrounded by props from the 50s they were asked to act as if it was actually 1959. They watched films, listened to music and discussed news events of the time – all as if these things were new and happening right in the present.

Understandably, Prof. Langer herself had doubts. "You have to understand when these people came to see if they could be in the study and they were walking down the hall to get to my office, they looked like they were on their last legs, so much so that I said to my students 'why are we doing this? It's too risky'."

As the week went by, Prof Langer began to notice that they were walking faster and their confidence had improved. One man decided to do without his walking stick. At the end of the week they played an impromptu game of 'touch' American football.

Physiological and psychological measurements were taken both before and after the week and found the men improved across the board. Their gait, dexterity, arthritis, speed of movement, cognitive abilities and their memory were all measurably improved. Their blood pressure dropped and, even more surprisingly, their eyesight and hearing got better.

How's that for the power of the mind-body connection!

In another example of Prof. Langer's research, she took 84 hotel housekeeping staff and told one group of them that the work they did (cleaning hotel rooms) was good exercise. She told the control group nothing. Four weeks later there were no changes to the control group, however, the test group had decreased in weight, blood pressure, body fat, waist-to-hip ratio, and body mass index. Their work hadn't changed, so it seems that some new thinking or belief in the hotel workers had been enough to change their bodies.

This aligns with the latest research[1] on stress that shows that stress only has a negative impact on your body if you think it does. It's the stress about having stress, not the original stressy Thought!

A study[2] presented to the European Society of Human Reproduction and Embryology conference in Berlin in July of 2004, demonstrated how hypnosis can improve fertility and effectively double the success of IVF treatments. The study of 185 women found that 28% of the women who were hypnotised for the IVF treatment became pregnant, compared to 14% of the women in the control group. This led to Professor Levitas studying hypnosis, having used medications such as tranquillisers in previous studies; none of them worked as well as hypnosis.

So you have more control over your body than you may think!

1. Keller A, Litzelman K, Wisk LE, Maddox T, Cheng ER, Creswell PD, Witt WP., *Does the perception that stress affects health matter?* The association with health and mortality, Health Psychol. 2012 Sep;31(5):677-84., 2011

2. Levitas E, Parmet A, Lunenfeld E, Bentov Y, Burnstein E, Friger M, Potaschnik G. *Impact of hypnosis during embryo transfer on the outcome of vitro fertilisation-embryo transfer: a case-control study.* Fertility & Sterility. 2006; 85(5), 1406-1408

37

❖

Thinking affects our biology

Y ou have probably heard of a placebo or the placebo effect. A placebo is a dummy drug used in medical trials in order to test the effectiveness of new drugs. Placebos do not contain any healing chemicals, they are typically something like sugar pills or water. They are given to some of the participants in the trial of new drugs. Placebos are supposed to have no effect, to act as a baseline to judge the success of the new drug. They are not supposed to heal but, the thing is, they frequently do because the patients in the trial believe they are taking the new effective drug. Their belief heals them.

The effectiveness of placebos very much depends upon the illness, the nature of the medical trial and the way in which they are prescribed. The biggest factor is the patients' belief that they will get better. 35% is often quoted as the effectiveness of placebos but it can be as low as 10% or as high as 100%[1].

In traditional western medicine there is an increasing interest in 'the placebo effect'. More and more research is taking place to understand how it works. New technology, such as brain scanners, is providing scientists with further insight into how placebos work. Research now shows that when we take a placebo, believing it to be an effective drug, the brain responds in a similar way as if we are taking the actual drug. The brain triggers the production of a natural chemical that is tailor-made to combat the illness.

This was first proven in 1978 where scientists at the University of California showed placebo painkillers worked because the brain was producing its own painkilling chemical (analgesics).

So, no longer can the placebo effect be dismissed as being 'all in the mind'. When you believe something, chemicals are produced in your brain, carrying out what you believe should happen. Your mind affects your body biologically.

In a study carried out by the Learner Institute in 2003[2] a group of volunteers visualised exercising their little finger over a period of 12 weeks (for 15 minutes per day, 5 days per week). They were encouraged to imagine how it would feel as they visualised the exercises. Their change in muscle strength was compared to a control group that didn't do any visualisations or physical exercises. By the end of the 12-week study, the muscle strength of the group visualising had improved by 35% and continued improving to 40% four weeks after the study and training had ended. So you can get fitter without lifting a finger!

In his book The Biology of Belief[3], cellular biologist Bruce Lipton explains how thinking can affect our body down the cellular and DNA level, in a fairly new area of biology called epigenetics.

I have had clients that don't ovulate on one side or in the past during IVF only harvested a small number of high-quality eggs. Once we work together, which includes using visualisation as a way of harnessing this mind-body link, they often experience physiological changes such as ovulation on both sides and harvesting a higher number of good quality eggs. One client used to picture in her mind healthy eggs as green dots and other eggs as red dots. I created a hypnosis visualisation recording for her to listen to helping her imagine more and more green dots. On her next (4th) IVF cycle she harvested twice the number of good quality eggs than any other cycle (and the IVF was successful!). Was it the only thing that made the difference? Probably not. But she believed it was a significant factor to her success.

In 1957 a patient, Mr Wright[4] who had terminal cancer was given a life expectancy of two weeks by his doctor, Bruno Klopfer. His only medication was oxygen to breathe and a sedative to help him on his way. However, Mr Wright had enormous faith in a new miracle drug (Krebiozen) that was being tested in the clinic he was in. He didn't qualify for the programme because his condition was too serious. He begged so hard that his doctor gave him a single injection of Krebiozen. His doctor then noted that 'the tumour masses had melted like snowballs on a hot stove." In three days they were half their original size and he was walking around the ward chatting happily.

Mr Wright was symptom-free for two months until he read in the newspaper that Krebiozen was worthless at treating cancer. Mr Wright began to lose faith in his last hope; he relapsed to his original state and was re-admitted to the hospital.

With nothing to lose, his doctor assured him that the first batch had deteriorated rapidly in the bottles and a new super-refined double-strength product was due to arrive the next day. The next day what Mr Wright actually received was an injection of salt water. Once again he was symptom-free for two months. Then the headlines again proclaimed that the national tests of the drug had proved it to be worthless in the treatment of cancer. With his faith now gone Mr Wright relapsed and died two days later.

---

1. Hamilton, D. *Your Mind Can Heal Your Body*. US, Hay House Inc; 2010. p31–42.

2. Ranganathan V, Siemionow V, Liu J, Sahgal V, Yue G. *From mental power to muscle power – gaining strength by using the mind, Neuropsychologia.* 2004;42: 944–956

3. Lipton B, *The Biology of Belief,* US, Hay House Inc; 2005.

4. Klopfer B, *Journal of Projective Techniques.* 1957;21: 331–340.

38

❖

What is visualisation?

Y ou may have heard of the term 'visualisation' but may not be sure exactly what it is or how you do it.

Visualisation is imagining something in your mind. If I were to ask you what the colour of your front door was, you will probably make a very quick mental image of the door before answering. Sometimes this happens so quickly we fail to recognise it. That's visualisation. Creating a mental image or getting a mental depiction of something usually through images (hence the term visualisation) though it can also involve feelings, sounds, a vague 'sense' rather than a clear photographic image or high definition film.

Sometimes the term 'visualisation' can put people off because they worry that they don't have the ability to create detailed visual images. That's OK. It doesn't mean you cannot visualise. Some people have a clearer image than others. Some people have a vague image or get a 'sense' of the thing they are visualising. All of those can be just as effective.

When you 'visualise' playing the piano you are imagining the keyboard, the finger movements, how it feels and perhaps even the sounds that go with it. All these aspects of the imagination are being registered by the brain and it is responding as if you really were playing the piano. This powerful phenomenon can help you achieve those things you most want in your life including, getting pregnant.

Your unconscious mind controls all your bodily functions. When you cut yourself your body heals. That process is controlled by your unconscious mind. However, sometimes it can benefit from some guidance to guide it to do what we want it to do.

Through visualisation, you can access and influence your unconscious mind to make changes in the body as if what you were imagining were real. Visualisation is one of the tools used by hypnotherapists and it can also be used as a form of self-hypnosis.

In 1994, Harvard scientists taught a simple 5-fingered combination of piano notes to a group of volunteers using all their fingers. They were instructed to play it over and over again for two hours a day, for five consecutive days. Another group of volunteers didn't actually play the notes, but just imagined playing them for the same period, two hours a day for five consecutive days. Whilst doing this they also imagined hearing the notes. The brain scans taken over the 5 days show the changes to the brain were almost identical for each group.

The brain can't tell the difference between imagination and reality!

Not only was there no difference in the brain's response, there was a significant effect on their later physical performance. After five days the ability (measured by the number of mistakes made) of the group that carried out mental practice only was the same as those that had been physically practising for three days. After just two hours of physical practice, they caught up and were at the same level as those that had been practising two hours a day for the full five days.

I regularly use visualisation for physical healing. I believe it has assisted in a range of things, from allergies to recovery from sports injuries and illnesses. A specific example is that my family went down with a stomach bug and my wife and son took three to four days to get better, however, I recovered within 24hrs and was by no means as ill as they were. I visualised my immune system being strong and fighting any bugs within me. I have seen the same powerful response from my clients.

Visualisation techniques can be utilised alongside medical interventions or other natural holistic approaches (such as acupuncture) to greatly improve the likelihood of your getting pregnant and maintaining a strong and healthy pregnancy. The mind and body are one system. So often we are focussed on the body and are not aware of the power of the mind-body connection.

Dr David Hamilton is a scientist who has studied the power of the mind and visualisation for many years. He used to work for a pharmaceutical company. When they tested new drugs they compared it to sugar pills, the placebo. He was amazed by how well placebos often performed. Of course, the company had no invested interest to explore this further so in his spare time he studied the placebo effect and mind-body link fervently. In the end, he left the company and has dedicated his life to helping people understand the power of their mind for their health and well-being. David coined a term 'feelingisation'[1]. He too believes it doesn't have to be limited to images. In fact the more you play with your imagination and the feelings you imagine you would feel, whilst imagining your body is doing what you want it to do, the more effective it can be.

---

1. Hamilton D. *Your Mind Can Heal Your Body*. US, Hay House Inc; 2008.

39

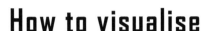

How to visualise

So if visualisation is creating a mental image or getting a mental depiction of something, why do we need to learn how to do it? I have included this chapter because some people say they cannot visualise or find it hard to visualise. I think everyone can visualise but if you find it doesn't come easy to you like most things, it gets easier with practice. The mental images are not a pre-requisite for success. As per the previous chapter, getting a sense or feeling of something can be just as effective.

Whether recalling an image from the past or creating an image of something you want in the future, it can be a matter of honing the same technique. Below is an exercise you can use to grow your ability to create mental images. The more you practise the easier you will find it. You may then find it easier to get into visualising/sensing your body doing what you want it to do for you to get pregnant.

Visualisation Exercise

Start with the first step and practise each step until you are confident with it before moving on to the next one. Perhaps spend a week practising for five minutes twice a day and you may begin to notice it getting easier and/or the images getting more vivid.

1. Picture a matchbox. Whatever comes to mind, however vague or brief, is visualisation. The more you do it the

clearer it can become or the longer you will be able to hold the picture in your mind.

2. Now start to notice more and more detail. If it had a colour what colour would it be? Imagine a picture on the front. Spend some time noticing more and more about the matchbox, you may become aware of more detail. Play with your imagination.

3. Can you change the colour of the matchbox? Practise changing it from colour to colour.

4. Can you rotate the matchbox so it is standing on its end or side, or perhaps turn it upside down.

5. What other creative things can you do with this match-box in your mind? If you imagine opening it, I wonder if you will find matches inside.

6. Can you imagine what it feels like against your skin? How it would feel as you move it around, perhaps feeling the edges or the texture of the striking strip. What would it feel like if the striking area was sandpaper found on some brands of matches?

What to visualise

A common question I am asked is what to visualise. There is no magic formula. There is, in fact, no right or wrong. The most powerful visualisation is when it utilises your own imagination and unconscious mind which is unique to you rather than you being told what to visualise. It's getting a sense of what you think could benefit your body the most. You may imagine your body ovulating. Or, if having IVF, your body welcoming the embryo and nurturing it or harvesting high-quality eggs. It could be any of these, all of these or something different, perhaps hormones being in a healthy balance.

So what you visualise comes from your instinct, intuition as to what is right for you, at this stage of the process. How you visualise it is also more powerful when it comes from you. Again there is no right or wrong. Some people may visualise these things in a more biological way, others have more symbolic or metaphoric images, it really doesn't matter.

When I visualise my body dealing with a virus I sometimes see the 1980s arcade game character 'Pacman' eating the 'dots' of virus in my body, at other times I imagine my immune system being strengthened with the arrival of the cavalry, an army of Stormtroopers (but working for the goodies!) bringing power and strength that virus can't compete with. Perhaps I played too many computer games and watched too many films in my youth!

I have had clients imagining a more anatomically correct image, but it really doesn't matter what imagery you use. A key thing is to be aware of the emotions that go along with it so you sink deeper into the visualisation as if it were real. Feel how you would feel knowing this was taking place inside you as you imagine it.

I recommend you start by visualising what you want your body to be doing in this moment. Connect with it in this moment and imagine what you want it to be doing right now. Perhaps hormones balancing, your body working with the medication, your body preparing for ovulation. Then as you get into it, begin to imagine that process playing out in the future. What happens from here? Perhaps the embryo being welcomed by the uterus lining. Embracing it and over time seeing it being more and more embedded. Start with where you are now and then imagine the process as you want it to play out. This gives your unconscious mind clear instructions for the here and now and a direction to head towards.

Being guided through a visualisation and including a time of relaxation beforehand can make it far more powerful because it enables you to enter the visualisation in a more vivid way by getting your conscious (logical, thinking) mind out of the way. I use an mp3 audio track I have created for my healing visualisation. If you want to explore using a fertility hypnosis programme that utilises visualisation wrapped around powerful hypnotic language, take a look at the hypnosis programmes you can download from my website www.thefertilemind.net.

When to visualise?

Another common question is how long do I visualise for and how frequently? Again there is no right or wrong but if you wanted some suggestions to get you started, I recommend you sit down and spend 3-5 minutes visualising twice a day. You may be surprised as time goes by how the images come to mind at other times of the day reminding you that your unconscious mind is processing and doing what you have been guiding it to do.

Part 4

The male perspective

40

❖

The male perspective

My wife and I had a 10-year journey of infertility, involving both female and male infertility. I wouldn't wish a 10-year infertility experience on anyone, however, I can look back and be so thankful for some of the things I learned about myself, life and relationships that have made a huge positive difference to my life, and in the end my fertility.

We're not given a manual on how to be a man or how to do relationships. Often we learn to see how our parents interact and live out life. My dad was a lovely man, very kind, but was emasculated by my mum who was dominant. It's only through our fertility journey and my commitment to knowing how to best support my wife I began to learn what it means to be and relate to the feminine. What I learned surprised me but has changed my life for the better forever. My wish is for other men to know some of this for their own life, for their relationship, for their happiness and well-being.

I encourage you to read these chapters for men in this section and, if you want to really know how to best support your partner, read the rest of the relationship section. It's the manual I wish I had.

41

What you may be experiencing

I experienced a whole range of emotions on our fertility journey. It took me a while to recognise them because habitually I ignored or buried feelings. Here I want to share some of the experiences I had on my journey that I know other men have. I do this so you can know you're not alone, or bad or wrong for feeling such feelings. It's called being human!

Responsible

You may feel responsible for being the 'strong one' in the relationship. For being there for your partner. For not showing any emotion because you don't want to burden her any more than she is already. You want to make this journey as easy for her as possible.

I was not aware that by doing this I was making it worse. My wife felt alone on the journey because I wasn't sharing my emotions. I didn't recognise that that's how women want to connect – emotionally. She wanted to *feel* us being in it together. To understand how I felt too and for her feelings to be understood by me. That doesn't mean we have to feel the same thing, it means understanding how each other feels about the situation.

Confused

You may be confused as to how to best support your partner in all this. When you see her upset you want to make her feel better.

When you try it often ends up making it worse!

This is a masculine and feminine thing. Often men do not know how to deal with feminine energy, feminine emotion. They don't like to see their woman feeling upset or in pain as they want to fix it, they want to change it.

However, women just want to be seen, felt, heard. They don't want their man to change it, they want them to understand it. They want their man to hold a space for that emotion without any judgment or evaluation of it. For them to feel OK for feeling it. They don't want their man to fix their problem, they can fix their own problems, they want to feel understood in the problem. So many men don't understand this. I didn't until the midst of our fertility journey. Don't get me wrong, I still don't always get it right! But I am far more aware of the error of my ways when I fall in to trying to fix how my wife is feeling.

Nothing

You may think you're not feeling anything. Now technically that isn't true but that may be your experience. Men often have a very distant relationship with emotions for various reasons. Culturally men are brought up in a society that says big boys don't cry. Men are bombarded with messages that being a man means not being emotional. That being emotional is a weakness. Consciously they may know that's not true. But unconsciously that is the message they have been getting from a very young age.

There may be other reasons why men have a distance relationship with emotions. Perhaps there was stuff that happened in their childhood that hasn't been processed or acknowledged; it's easy just to bury it as a protection mechanism. However, this can often result in burying all emotions. This was certainly my experience.

In times of stress men go to their 'nothing' place in their head. In times of stress women want to talk about how they feel about it. Nothing infuriates a woman more than seeing a man doing 'nothing' (e.g. channel surfing, playing computer games). Nothing infuriates a man more than a woman wanting to talk about something 'over and over' when they don't see it as actually helping solve the problem. Neither is right or wrong. Just different.

Inadequacy

If you have fertility problems yourself, as I did, you may be judging yourself to be less of a man in some way. You may subconsciously think that part of your core manliness is missing, that compared to other men you are less of a man because you cannot father children. You may be consciously aware of this or it may be an under-current you haven't fully acknowledged, or want to acknowledge. You may feel inadequate as a husband if you judge it to be your fault that you cannot have children.

I could see my wife was just born to parent. She was a natural. We had children and young people in our lives and she loved being around them and they loved being around her. And (after her own eight-year fertility journey) I was the reason she couldn't be a parent, the thing she wanted most in life.

Fear

If you judge yourself as the cause of the problem, part of you may be fearful that ultimately your partner may leave you. That one day her desire to have children will be stronger than the relationship. This sounds quite extreme and many can never imagine it happening but fear is the misuse of imagination. It runs away with itself and loses a sense of perspective and reality. It's plausible in your mind. It doesn't mean you think there is anything wrong with the relationship now or that you don't love her, or she doesn't love you. It is part of you is racing ahead to some time in the future and seeing her having a change of heart, that her desire to have children is too strong to ignore at whatever cost. This fearful thinking is natural and doesn't mean she doesn't love you and want to be with you. It really is the mis-use of imagination. Nothing can predict the future, not even your thinking.

42

Men and the emotional rollercoaster

One of the biggest things that I have benefited from as a result of our fertility journey, and was probably the catalyst to us conceiving naturally against all odds, was the change in my relationship with emotions.

Infertility is known as an emotional rollercoaster. A Harvard University study[1] demonstrates the stress levels of women experiencing infertility can be equivalent to those with AIDS, cancer and heart disease. And no one tells them just to relax! The study didn't test the stress levels of men but I imagine they would be similar albeit more hidden.

Before our infertility journey, and during the majority of it, I had a very distant relationship with emotions. Subconsciously I avoided strong emotions. I avoided conflict and negative emotions because I thought they were unhelpful and destructive. During our fertility journey, I also tried to be the strong one. I didn't want to burden my wife with my stuff, she had enough to deal with as it was. Little did I know all of this was both impacting my own fertility but also pushing our relationship to breaking point.

As boys and men, we are bombarded with messages about what it means to be a man. This can come both unconsciously and consciously from our fathers but also media and society as a whole. The typical male idols of kids are deemed to be strong, powerful and rarely express real deep emotion. In the school playground, it is survival of the fittest and you daren't show any weakness. So we can learn that expressing emotions can be a weakness.

I grew up in an environment where there was a lot of conflict. I learnt to keep my head down. To retreat into my head as it was safer there. I couldn't get emotionally hurt, disappointed or let down.

Thinking v Feeling

The thinking we learn about ourselves and life as we grow up can create thought habits that unconsciously shape our perception and experience of life as an adult. I wasn't aware of this until our infertility journey. It is very unconscious. In the past, my wife had complained that she found me being in my head so much hard but I didn't realise how much of a problem it was creating. Eight years into our infertility journey, at our lowest point, my wife told me she felt alone on the journey. I was shocked. I went to every appointment. We talked about things. So I thought. She told me she had no idea how I felt about things. At the same time, she was going through the grieving process. Grieving the possibility of not having children. I would say I was angry but found it hard to actually feel it. This highlighted to me my unconscious distant relationship with emotions.

Completely out of character, I took myself on a silent retreat. I had an urge just to be. To be without any distraction of work, the internet, life. I realised I kept myself busy physically and mentally to avoid feeling. This was time to just be and feel whatever came up. It was a powerful experience. I cried. I got angry. I felt sad. I found a sense of peace. But ultimately what I learnt was feelings were not scary and I didn't have to avoid them.

What is an emotion?

Since then my exploration of feelings has helped me understand the true nature of emotions. We think we are feeling life and circumstances. We think we are angry because someone just let us down, or once again the traffic made us late for an important meeting. The thing is, nothing has the power to make us feel anything. 100% of our human experience comes from thought. We live and experience our perception of reality. If it was the circumstances that made us feel something we would feel the same feeling until the circumstances changed. But it doesn't work like that. Some days feel better than others even though the circumstances have not changed. If it was the circumstances that caused our experience then everyone who had the same circumstances would have the same experience of it. But again, it doesn't work like that. Everyone has their own unique experience created by thought, their own perception of the situation.

The more we understand that everything we experience comes from thought in this moment the more we realise we don't need to be scared of it. The more we resist our emotions, or try and change them, they don't move on. They either hang around, get stronger or worse we bury them and internalise them. Little did I know the damage I was doing to my relationship and my fertility by doing that.

Life beyond fear

When I stopped trying to bury my emotions, when I was no longer scared of feeling them, I felt like less of a victim in life. A few months after this realisation and experience my wife got pregnant naturally against all odds. My fertility had improved dramatically without me trying to improve it. In fact, I'd given up trying to improve it because everything I was doing to try and improve it actually made it worse. This was because my buried fear and anger were doing more damage than anything I was doing to improve my fertility. This was the thing that made the difference in our fertility journey.

When I began to understand the true nature of feelings two things happened that transformed our relationship. Firstly, I felt more able to understand how I felt in any given moment and thus express that to my wife. Instead of genuinely not knowing how I felt and saying my usual 'I don't know' when she asked how I felt or saying what I thought instead of how I felt (there's a big difference). Women like to connect with others on an emotional level. To understand how they are feeling. And to be understood emotionally as well. They feel united, loved and understood when that happens.

Secondly, I was able to help her feel more understood. Men communicate information as and when required. They share a problem because they are looking for a solution. Women communicate to be understood. Women want to be seen, felt and heard. Women communicate a problem or a feeling to be understood in it. This difference can come to the fore at times of stress, such as infertility. Habitually when my wife was upset I would try and make her feel better, or provide a solution. This seemed to make things worse! I got to the stage where I just didn't know what to do. Part of me felt scared of her emotion. This left her feeling unloved, lonely and misunderstood. This creates a distance in a relationship.

I began to realise what she wanted was for me to hold a space for her to express her emotion without any judgment or evaluation. Without trying to fix or change it. The more I understood emotion wasn't coming from the circumstances, that she may think it's my fault she's angry but knowing it's 100% thought, I no longer became scared of it. I could see it for what it is, her experience in this moment, it will probably be different in a few moments time. Don't get me wrong, there are times I still make the mistake and think it's personal, that she is having a go at me. In those times it's easy to get defensive and the exchange can become less than loving.

Getting comfortable with feeling uncomfortable

Starting to be more aware of your emotions, allowing them and even expressing them can feel unfamiliar or even uncomfortable. The more you understand the true nature of an emotion, that it's thought in the moment, the less scared of it you become. Also, you become more able to express how you feel. The emotion doesn't get stuck, it flows from you. The sense of flow comes into your life (and your body) as well as a deeper sense of connection with your partner even in the toughest of times. Because it's in those times we need to feel loved and understood more than anything.

---

1. Domar AD, et al. *The Psychological Impact of Infertility: A Comparison with Patients with Other Medical Conditions.* Journal of Psychosomatic Obstetrics and Gynaecology 14 Suppl.: pp45–52, 1993.

43

❖

Emotions

"And numbing vulnerability is especially debilitating because it doesn't just deaden the pain of our difficult experiences; numbing vulnerability also dulls our experiences of love, joy, belonging, creativity, and empathy. We can't selectively numb emotion. Numb the dark and you numb the light." Brené Brown

Emotions were an alien concept to me for various reasons. One is that there were painful emotions from the past that I wanted to bury so subconsciously I thought emotions are best avoided. I was totally unaware that I was doing this using my thinking/being my head as a way of protecting myself from being hurt emotionally.

Another reason was being raised in a society with an undercurrent of 'big boys don't cry'. I see the same relationship with emotions in many of my male clients. Boys learn to be men by taking the messages about what it means to be a man through parents, older siblings, peers, teachers, TV shows, action films, commercials, men in positions of leadership, whether scout leaders or PMs. Many of these messages encourage boys to be competitive, focus on material success, think, be physically strong and suppress any vulnerability or emotions.

A study[1] in the US looked at the attributes associated with masculinity. It identified that people associated the following:

- Winning: "In general, I will do anything to win"
- Emotional Control: "I tend to keep my feelings to myself"
- Risk-Taking: "Taking dangerous risks helps me to prove myself"
- Violence: "Sometimes violent action is necessary"
- Dominance: "I should be in charge"
- Playboy: "If I could, I would frequently change sexual partners"
- Self-Reliance: "Asking for help is a sign of failure"
- Primacy of Work: "My work is the most important part of my life"
- Power Over Women: "In general, I control the women in my life"
- Disdain for Homosexuals: "I make sure that people think that I am heterosexual"
- Pursuit of Status: "It feels good to be important."

When boys do express emotions or vulnerability it often leads to them being teased or ridiculed. Is not uncommon for men to think that showing emotions or being vulnerable is a sign of weakness.

For these reasons, whether it is childhood emotions being buried as a protection mechanism or being brought up with the message that emotions are a sign of weakness, many men find it hard to identify their feelings let alone express them.

We all have feelings, it is just that some of us find it easier to be aware and in tune with them than others. Often men say they find it difficult to be in tune with their feelings…or do they…?

I remember a European Cup Final. Chelsea was losing 1-0 with a few minutes to go. They scored an equaliser in the dying minutes that took the game to extra time – you could feel the relief of the supporters across the country wave through the TV set. 30 minutes of extra time, a tense waiting game. Then came the penalty shoot-out. The tension went up a notch, this was it, make or break. Chelsea was down and looking like this was it but then they turned things around and when things looked so hopeless only a few minutes previously, they became European Champions.

I would like to suggest 99% of the male supporters went through a rollercoaster of emotions from hope, joy, despair, anger, fear, sadness, anxiety… Of course, nothing the same magnitude as infertility, however, I believe many of these men are the same men who say they don't feel their feelings!

Brené Brown is a research professor at the University of Houston, Graduate College of Social Work. She has spent the past decade studying vulnerability, courage, worthiness, and shame.

Her 2010 TEDx Houston talk on the power of vulnerability is one of the most watched talks on TED.com with over 7 million views. Her book *Daring Greatly* is an excellent exploration of vulnerability and how the messages from society around emotions and shame prevent us from living the inspired life we crave. In the book[2] Brené summarises her research on men and vulnerability as.

"When I asked men to define shame, here's what I heard:

- Shame is failure. At work. On the football field. In your marriage. In bed. With money. With your children. It doesn't matter—shame is failure.
- Shame is being wrong. Not doing it wrong, but being wrong.
- Shame is a sense of being defective.
- Shame happens when people think you're soft. It's degrading and shaming to be seen as anything but tough.
- Revealing any weakness is shaming. Basically, shame is weakness.

- Showing fear is shameful. You can't show fear. You can't be afraid—no matter what.
- Shame is being seen as "the guy you can shove up against the lockers."
- Our worst fear is being criticised or ridiculed—either one of these is extremely shaming.

Basically, men live under the pressure of one unrelenting message: Do not be perceived as weak."

Brené Brown, *Daring Greatly*, p91

The thing is, this protection mechanism that men have to prevent them from 'being perceived as weak' actually prevents us from having the experiences in life we aspire to have. To feel loved deeply and passionately by our partner. To experience the highs and lows of life, just like the football match. This protection mechanism means we flatline through life. Being 'OK' but not really living and engaged in life and thus experiencing the joys it can bring.

I lived my life that way for many years (decades). It felt safe but at the same time, it stopped me being truly happy. It also drove a wedge between me and my wife.

Numbing our vulnerability doesn't just prevent us from feeling difficult feelings, it also numbs the experiences of joy, happiness, inspiration and love. You can't selectively numb the 'negative' emotions and just feel the 'positive ones'. You end up flat-lining through life. It's better to be alive to life than dead to life.

---

1. Mahalik J R, Locke BD, Ludlow L, Diemer M, Scott RPJ, Gottfried M, Freitas G. *Development of the Conformity to Masculine Norms Inventory. Psychology of Men and Masculinity*, 2003;4: 3–25.

2. Brown B. *Daring Greatly*. US, Portfolio Penguin; 2013. p91.

44

❖

Being the strong one

After eight years of being married and many years of infertility, my wife one day told me that she felt alone on the journey. I was really surprised by this. I attended all the appointments. We talked about the things and made the decisions together. How was it that she felt alone?

She told me that she didn't feel united on the journey. Emotionally united. She said she didn't understand what was going on within me, within my head. She said she didn't know how I felt about things. I must admit this had been quite a common complaint in our relationship, that I lived in my head and that I wasn't present.

I can see how I lived in my head for two reasons. One was I generally didn't know how I felt at any given point. I really wasn't aware of my emotions let alone able to articulate them. The second reason was I thought I needed to be the strong one, to be strong for her and not allow my feelings to be an additional burden for her.

It turns out that's not what she wanted.

She wanted to know how I felt. She wanted me to understand how she felt. It is this sharing and understanding at an emotional level that enables a woman to feel united with her man.

This can be a very alien concept for a man. Emotions can be a very alien for a man.

All we want to do is help, support and love our woman. The problem is no-one has ever taught us how to do that. No-one has given us the manual for women! And like-wise no-one gave them the manual for men.

I never understood why so many times I tried to help my wife somehow what I said made things worse. It turns out they don't want us to make them feel better or to fix their problems. They want to feel understood. And they want to understand how we feel. Not what we think.

There can be a cultural undertone of men being the 'provider', being the strong one to protect and look after our partner. Whilst it is true that women want their men to be strong, to be able to create a container that can contain their emotions, without judgement and without trying to fix or change it, this can take strength of character. I for one used to psychologically run away from my wife's strong emotions, not knowing how to help her as it seemed most things I tried in the past made it worse. However, that's because I judged her feelings as 'bad' and tried to change it, wanting her to feel OK.

Women's emotions are like a river, they flow. When they flow they move on. Like a river needs a bank to allow the flow, female emotions need a container to allow them to flow. Without a safe container, they can get stuck. It's our job to create that container. Space where they can express themselves without feeling judged and without anyone trying to change/fix the emotion. When we try to fix it all they hear is they are wrong for feeling it in the first place. Imagine they just need to vomit out these emotions. Our job is to hold the bucket. When they are done fresh emotions will come in automatically. We don't need to fix them. Listen, validate and empathise but don't fix!

Women don't just want their men to create such a container, they also want their men to be real, be vulnerable, to share their feelings. Men too often see expressing emotions as a weakness. Society creates a perception that 'big boys don't cry'. Well, that's not true. That is an adolescent form of male energy depicted by society and the media. Repressing our emotions leads to men being either aggressive and angry or passive 'Mr Nice Guys' (people pleasers). Women don't want Mr Nice Guy.

She wants you to be able to cry. She wants you to be real. To be vulnerable.

So she wants you to be able to hold a space for her emotions and share your emotions. What does this mean in practice? Where's the Hayne's manual to know how to actually do this? Read the relationship chapters of this book and you'll find step by step guides for you!

Part 5

Your thinking & relationships

45

❖

Fertility and relationships

The stress of infertility can put a strain on the best of relationships. My wife and I know firsthand of the impact it can have on a relationship. I am thankful for some of the things I learned about myself, women and relationships that I am indebted to.

Dealing with infertility can be tough enough on its own. Unfortunately, a study found that the pain of infertility can cause even more pain and heartache. Couples who didn't have a baby after fertility treatments were more likely to break up.

The study[1], which was published in the journal Acta Obstetricia et Gynecologica Scandinavica, Danish researchers tracked 47,515 women who were evaluated for infertility over 12 years. After the 12-year follow-up period, it turns out that the women who didn't have a child were up to three times more likely to have divorced or ended their relationship with the person they were with at the time of the study than the women who gave birth.

Another study[2] by Cardiff University showed that marital distress in women can increase the number of treatment cycles required for pregnancy. Although the study was only tracking women undergoing fertility treatment, you can bet your bottom dollar it will affect natural conception as well.

So it can become a double bind. Infertility can cause stress in a relationship which in turn can impact your fertility!

The good news is that you can break that cycle. And this is what this section is all about.

What causes relationship distress is not the circumstances of your fertility, whether you have a baby yet not. It is a lack of connection, understanding and feeling loved.

It is very easy to forget we all live in separate realities created by thought. We think the way we see things is the most logical and correct way. We get frustrated when others don't see things our way, or take the time to understand how we feel and see things. How we experience things in this moment is shaped by life experiences (mainly childhood). Gender can also have a large impact on our perception of reality. Men and women often think differently, we are wired differently. In essence, men forget women are not like them and visa-versa, and we think the world would be an easier (and better?) place if they were!

In this section, we are going to dissect some of the misunderstandings and lazy communication that is the cause of most relationship distress. To find new ways of connecting with each other. To communicate in a way that results in us feeling more loved, understood and united. For me, this is the glue in any relationship.

---

1. Kjaer T, Albieri V, Jensen A, Kjaer SK, Johansen C, Dalton SO. *Divorce or end of cohabitation among Danish women evaluated for fertility problems*, Acta Obstet Gynecol Scand. 2014;93(3):269-76.

2. Boivin, Schmidt, *Infertility-related stress and treatment outcome*, Fertility and Sterility, 2005; 83 (6)

46

❖

The difference between men's and women's brains

In this chapter, I am going to use stereotypes which although largely may be true may not always be true. Stereotyping the differences between men and women can sometimes oversimplify the differences between the way people process information in their own minds. For example, there can be very wide differences in how a same-sex couple process information, it is not just down to gender differences. Some research shows there is very little difference between a man's and a woman's brain and the differences in how we express ourselves in life is largely cultural. Whether it's biological or cultural, in my experience there can be useful generalisations that can help a couple understand each other and communicate more effectively leading to feeling more loved and united.

One difference between men and women is in the way they communicate. Women tend to communicate to feel understood, to share how they are feeling so the other person can empathise and understand. This brings an emotional connection. Men, however, tend to communicate transactionally, communicating facts and information on a need-to-know basis. This is often why men don't understand how women can spend so long talking to their friends. It can also lead to frustration when women don't feel understood by their men.

Men compartmentalise things in their mind. Their mind is a like a mansion with many rooms. Each room has a purpose and function. You finish what you are doing in one room before going to another room to do something else. When men talk about a subject they stick to that subject and cannot see the connection to other subjects or issues. This may not be the case in an argument; when you think you are losing an argument it can be tempting for either partner to steer it on to a subject you think you can win! I'm particularly good at that!

Women, however, have an 'open plan' brain. Their brain is one big space which occupies everything in their life. Women's brains are a big ball of energy where everything is connected to everything. All driven by an energy called emotions. Which is why women tend to remember more things than men. The brain stores memories with emotions and thus recalls memories more easily when associated with an emotion.

These differences can be brought to the fore at times. Typically when a man is stressed they go into their 'nothing room' of their brain mansion to ponder. They want to be alone there. Women don't understand their 'nothing room'. It is empty. They go there to do nothing. Nothing drives a woman crazier than seeing her man doing nothing. A man can flick through all the channels of the TV not watching anything and that can drive a woman mad, but it's the man being in his nothing room.

Women can't go into a man's nothing room. No matter how much he loves you, you are not welcome there! If you did you would want to decorate it and make it 'something', when the whole point is it's a nothing room! This is the place a man unwinds and deals with stress. They don't want to talk about it. How many times have you asked your man what he's thinking about and he says 'nothing'. Women can't understand how men can think about 'nothing'.

If a woman is stressed she needs to talk about it otherwise her brain will explode with all the energy. It can often come out with great energy and emotion. Men often can't handle this and run away from it because they don't know how to handle it. They can't see how to fix it because in the past when they have tried it didn't work or even made it worse. Men only tell their problems to another man to get help and advice on how to fix it. Men often don't know what to say to their women in these situations. They cannot see they don't want solutions. They want to be seen, heard and understood. Not changed or fixed. They want their man to shut up and listen.

These and other differences in how individuals interact with the world and each other can be a common source of stress in any relationship, particularly on the emotional rollercoaster of infertility.

Understanding that there are differences in how we interact with life can be hugely beneficial. We can realise the way our partner's behaviour is not personal. Women can begin to under-stand his not talking is not because he doesn't care. And men can understand that women are not trying to drag them out of their cave kicking and screaming because they are trying to annoy them. Men and women who love each other want to help each other and offer each other their finest solution, however, it's often the solution that they would not want what their partner wants.

Our over-sensitive thinking can make our partner's behaviour about us, we make it personal so get hurt or offended rather than seeing a man/woman dealing with stress in the way that's natural to them.

So women, don't be afraid to leave him alone when he is stressed and in his nothing room.

Men, don't give solutions unless she has asked you for advice in writing, in triplicate, from her lawyer! Listen. Read the next chapter on listening.

Men often want their women to be more like a man. Women often want their men to be more like a woman. Well, some of the time. However when we recognise our differences, and it is our differences that we were first attracted to (the energy of the opposite sex), then we can begin to find ways of communicating more effectively with more love and understanding.

As I said at the beginning of the chapter, these differences are not necessarily male/female. To understand more about your personality types and how you interact as a couple I thoroughly recommend the book *Lovebirds* by Trevor Silvester.

47

❖

Listening

'You're not listening to me' was a common thing my wife used to say to me. I didn't understand back then what she meant. I had listened and I'd shared my thoughts on what she had said. Since then I've learned what she meant and can see clearly why she felt not listened to.

The role of a listener is to listen for the feeling their partner is communicating. The essence of what they are saying beyond their words. As a way of explaining this, let's pretend there are three ways of listening – this is a model for demonstration purposes, not absolute truth.

Busy Mind Listening

Let me call the first way of listening 'Busy Mind Listening'. This is when you are listening to someone and your mind wanders and you find yourself thinking about something very different. Perhaps your mind has gone on to what you have forgotten to do earlier or what you need to do next, and are not actually listening to what they are saying at all! We all do it from time to time.

Another example of busy mind listening are the times when you are still thinking about what you were thinking about before they starting talking. You haven't finished the conversation with yourself in your head before this real one had started. They had no idea you were so busy in your head and launched into a conversation when you perhaps weren't fully ready. It is tempting in these situations to think you can do both, hold on to what you were thinking about in your mind and still listen. You can make all the right noises and think you are paying attention to them, but you're not being fully present to them and you will miss what they are actually wanting you to hear.

Active Listening

Active Listening is when you are listening to someone but at the same time thinking about what you are going to say in response. Formulating your response in your mind as they talk. You think you've got what they've said and you have moved on to what to say next. You may be thinking of all the reasons why they are wrong, how they've misunderstood a situation. Or you may be thinking of all the things you want to say to affirm the person. Either way, you are not being fully present to what they are really trying to communicate. You think you know and you've stopped listening. You have assumed you know what it is they want you to hear and your attention has moved on to your response. You have listened from your model of the world without getting into theirs to really understand what they mean by their words.

Deep Listening

A third way would be to listen with a quiet mind, what I would call 'Deep Listening'. To be present to the person without anything on your mind. Listening like a video camera, not filtering what it does or doesn't take it. There is no filter. Not thinking about how to respond or what your mind is doing. Being totally present to them, with a sense of peace and calm within you. It's listening without filtering through your own thinking, beliefs and model of the world. When you do this you hear beyond the words. You hear what their infinite soul is communicating between the finite words of our language. You get an insight in to what they are really communicating. It's listening without judgement or evaluation. It's hearing them from their experience and model of the world, not yours. Deep listening through a connection beyond words. From this space, you have no urge to say anything unless you feel totally inspired to.

A Rabbi I know was asked by a member of his synagogue to visit his son who had mental health problems and had been sectioned. His son refused to speak to anyone. Not a word. He had totally closed down. The rabbi went to visit him and started speaking. He didn't expect a response but found himself speaking to fill the silence. After a few minutes, he stopped himself. He asked himself why he was speaking. He realised he was doing it out of habit and to fill the silence. He got quiet within himself and decided to only speak when he felt totally inspired to say something. They sat in silence for about half an hour. At the end of their time together the Rabbi thanked the young lad for their time together and said he had really enjoyed it. And he had. He felt a real sense of connection with him in their silence. I don't know what happened after this but I am sure if the rabbi kept doing that the young lad would have begun opening up to him.

You may be aware that when you talk to someone sometimes you feel more connected to them than other times. That feeling of connection is two people being fully present to each other. Nothing on their minds, just being in that moment together. Really understanding each other in that moment. That's when people feel really understood.

We are formless infinite souls trying to communicate with a limited number of words. Listen with a quiet mind and you'll connect to the soul in front of you and really hear what they are trying to communicate beyond their words.

48

It's all about me

When we are little children we interpret situations and circumstances in a different way than we do as adults as our emotional intelligence hasn't formed yet. We can't comprehend the idea that our parents and other adults around us have 'their stuff/issues'. If we don't feel fully loved or accepted by our parents we tend to think it is to do with us. We think it's our fault. We tend to think kids in the playground won't play with us because there's something wrong with us.

We are tribal beings. Our physical survival used to be dependent on being part of a tribe. There are three parts of our brain, the reptilian brain (all about basic survival of eating, breathing and staying alive), the mammalian brain (wanting to be part of the pack/loved) and the human brain (creativity, cognitive thinking). The mammalian part of our brain still operates with tribal/pack mentality. Scared of not being loved or wanted.

As a child part of us thinks our survival is dependant on the tribe being secure and our position in the tribe being secure. The mammalian part of our brain wants unconditional positive regard from our caregivers to know we are OK. The 'tribe' most influential to us is the family unit but we also have other 'tribes' such as friendship circles.

My mum suffered from anxiety, was very strict and had high expectations of me and my siblings. When she shouted at me

I didn't feel loved. So I worked out what I needed to do to feel more loved. Do the things that please her. Don't do the things that make her angry. Be the 'good' boy she wanted me to be. I misunderstood it wasn't about me, that I was OK and I am fully loved and lovable for who I am. I learnt unconsciously that I was OK if my Mum was OK. I started to develop Outside-In Thought.

There is nothing else we could have done as kids. We think what we need to think to best cope, survive and understand situations in order to continue to be an accepted member of the pack. As adults, we can look back at those situations and see how it wasn't our fault, however as kids in the situation we see it differently. Now we can look back and know our parents loved us unconditionally and they were doing the best they could with the resources they had available. The way our parents and teachers were is due to their own upbringing, thoughts and beliefs, it wasn't about us.

Even though we are no longer the children we were in the situation, the Outside-In thought we develop can become a thought habit. We unconsciously see our current situation through the lens of this thinking about ourselves and the life we developed as a child. A lens of Outside-In Thought through which we create our present experience.

As a result, we tend to make things about us.

The boss talks to you in an angry tone and you assume it is about you. You assume he is upset with you and something you have done or not done. When perhaps he has just had an argument with his wife on the phone before he came to speak to you. Who knows why he is angry but our thinking makes it about us. We text a friend and they don't respond within minutes and we assume they don't like us or we've upset them in some way.

Even if someone's emotion, e.g. anger, is being directed at us, it's not about us. Even if they think it's about us (that we make them angry) it's not about us. It feels like it is about us because out habitual thinking thinks it is. However, everyone lives in the experience of their thinking, their experience. Their feelings are being created by their thinking, not us, not what we have done or said. That's impossible, we don't have the power to make someone feel anything. In the same way, someone doesn't have the power to make us feeling anything. We all live in our perception of reality created by our thinking.

When we take it personally and make it about us, we can end up getting defensive, justifying why they shouldn't be angry at us because we don't want them to be angry at us, we want them to be OK with us, so we are an accepted member of the pack. We start to believe we are OK if they think we are OK.

It's not about you.

It's their stuff. Thought creating their experience.

You are OK regardless of their experience at this moment. You haven't caused their experience. They just think you have and you have no control over their thinking.

Don't make it about you.

49

❖

Sharing

"I feel alone on this journey." I was shocked to hear those words from my wife. I went to all the appointments and I thought we talked about things.

Have you noticed conversations at a party tend to go along the lines of someone shares a story or anecdote then someone else shares one from their life related to the first one? And so it goes on. It is kept at a very safe surface anecdotal level. There is rarely any deeper sharing or vulnerability unless it's between very good friends. Of course, a conversation with strangers at a party may not be the place to pour your heart out but it is an example of how in our culture we often keep conversations at a surface level and avoid being vulnerable and sharing something deeper of ourselves. This can even happen unconsciously in a relationship.

The depth of connection with someone can be related to the depth of our sharing with that person. The more open and vulnerable we are the more we are sharing of ourselves, the more we can be felt by the other person. We often share our thoughts about something but not how we feel about it. Our emotions share something more of ourselves, of our internal experience. What's really going on within us. Our partner craves to understand that, particularly women.

I found it difficult to share my feelings because I wasn't even aware of them myself. I had lived in my head, my bubble of

Outside-In Thought, for so long identifying and communicating my feelings was quite alien to me. It was an unconscious protection mechanism because as a child I felt disappointed when I reached out for love from my mum but didn't get it (in the form I expected or wanted). My being closed emotionally saddened my wife because she felt shut out from the true me.

I knew I had to do something about this if we wanted a relationship. Someone feeling lonely in a relationship is not sustainable.

I came across the idea of a 'feelings audit' as a way of helping people be more aware of their inner self and their feelings. A few times during the day (typically mid-morning, lunchtime, mid-afternoon and at the end of the day) I would check in with myself. I would review what had happened over the last few hours and how I had felt about it. Typically situations would happen and I may have an emotional response but it would be so fleeting or I wouldn't even be consciously aware of it because I was so accustomed to being tuned in to my thinking. This meant it was soon forgotten without me acknowledging it. Some people may say this is a good thing as it stops you getting caught up in emotions, however for me it was being blind to part of myself and not fully acknowledging the whole me. Part of me had decided emotions were a bad thing (growing up with a lot of conflicts) so I denied them. In doing so I wasn't fully allowing me to be me, express myself freely, recognise and have my needs met in situations. Emotions are not destructive, it's our relationship with them and resulting behaviour that can be destructive. Even burying emotions can be destructive and lead to passive aggression.

This audit helped me recognise the feelings I had throughout my day. Writing them down helped me remember them so

I could share more of 'me' when I talked about my day with my wife, instead of just saying 'it was fine'!

Gradually being aware of my feelings became more natural. We have feelings and they don't kill you, they are not something you have to avoid – who knew!! Avoiding feelings meant I 'flat-lined' through life. I avoided the not so enjoyable ones but at the same time, I was inadvertently avoiding the enjoyable ones!

The process of writing my feelings down also helped me tune in to them. I began to write more about situations to help me tune in to how I felt about it. When I wrote the sentence 'When I think of [situation] I feel…' I started writing having no idea what I was feeling. However, the rule is to keep the pen moving. Sometimes I would start by writing 'I don't know what to write' over and over and then out of the blue a well of emotion would come out and on to the page. It was like releasing a beach ball that was being held under the water. If felt like I was coming back into alignment and being fully connected to all aspects of me. It felt good. Having identified these feelings I was then able to share them with my wife which helped us create a deeper connection and understanding.

It is worth checking what we mean by feelings and whether we really are sharing a feeling and not a thought or judgement. We often say the words 'I feel…' but what follows is not a feeling. 'I feel angry' is a feeling. 'I feel ignored' is not a feeling, it is a judgement that someone is ignoring you. As a rule of thumb if you can say 'I am X' it is probably a feeling. If saying 'I am X ' doesn't make sense then it is probably not a feeling. E.g. 'I feel angry'. 'I am angry'. That works because anger is a feeling. 'I feel let down'. 'I am let down.' That doesn't work because it is a judgement, not an emotion. It is key to keep away from judgements because they can be taken personally and this does not create a container for deep sharing and connecting, it becomes about blame and whether someone is right or wrong. Feelings are neither good/bad/right or wrong, they are spontaneous Thought coming alive in our consciousness in any given moment.

50

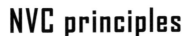

NVC principles

We can often be lazy with our communication and can be unaware of how powerful our words can be. Although we cannot control someone else's thinking and they have the response they have to what we say because of their thinking, if we are conscious of the language we use we can minimise the changes of the recipient hearing from their thinking and getting defensive and not really hearing what you are communicating.

Non Violent Communication (NVC) is a communication model created by the late American psychologist Marshell Rosenberg.

It is a simple but effective model that can help couples maximise the effectiveness of their communication so they can feel more understood and emotionally connected and united.

Marshall believes there isn't any situation in the world whether between individuals or countries (he worked with both!) that cannot be resolved and unity created when you communicate the needs behind an emotion.

It is a tool that recognises that no-one has the power to make us feel anything, we are living in the experience of our own thinking so our feelings are ours and not created by someone else. They didn't make us feel how we feel.

Observation

The first step in the non violent communication process is observation. Observation is about observing what is going on without including judgement or evaluation. It is separating observation and evaluation.

The purpose of excluding judgement and evaluation is that when we let these go we are more able to communicate ourselves purely, owning our experience, without others taking it personally or seeing it as a criticism.

For example, "you spent too much money" is a judgement, not an observation. "You spent £100 yesterday" is an observation. "You don't care about our treatment" is a judgement. "You haven't come with me to the last two appointments" is an observation.

Feelings

It is key that feelings are being expressed to create an understanding and connection between two people. Feelings are spontaneous internal reactions to Thought. They are neither good, bad, right or wrong. Nothing makes us feel anything because they are caused by Thought, not circumstances. We live in the experience of Thought in the moment.

In our communication, we often tell others they have 'made us' feel something. e.g. "You disappointed me by not coming to the last appointment". The thing is nothing has the power to make us feel anything. It is our Thought (perception) of a situation so we need to own the feeling. For example, "I was disappointed when you didn't come to the last appointment."

Another example of blaming an external circumstance or person for our feelings might be, "They cancelled our appointment and that really annoyed me!". However, more to be more accurate it is, "When they cancelled the appointment I felt annoyed because…[I am really keen to get moving with the treatment as I am worried we are running out of time]." Now we can begin to unravel what is really going on which creates understanding.

When we own feelings we are sharing something of ourselves. It is only when we do that honest communication can take place. When we blame others for our feelings then judgement, protection, barriers get in the way of creating unity and understanding.

When we own our feelings the listener is less likely to hear judgements and criticism which enables a more positive and constructive dialogue.

Needs

What is often behind our negative emotions are needs that are not being met. Being able to identify and articulate the need behind a feeling can deepen each other's understanding of a situation and can then lead to a way forward together. It makes sense that if we can communicate our needs we are more likely to have them met!

"I feel disappointed that you didn't come to the last appointment because I have a need to feel like we are on this journey together every step of the way."

The thing is we live in a society that says our experience moment to moment is created by external factors, an 'outside-in' approach to life. Marketing says 'buy this and you will feel x'. When we feel something we look for the external reason and this can lead to blaming others for the feeling.

What can be more constructive is looking within, because that is where the feeling originates from. Look within to see what need is not being met behind that feeling.

Requests

The fourth step of the NVC process is to make a request to the other person that can enrich your lives. It can be more effective if the request states what we want, not what we don't want, and is succinct and clear.

It is also key that it is a request and not a demand! When people hear demands they have one of two response: submit or rebel. The listener's ability to be compassionate and seek the mutual understanding and unity is diminished. Requests are heard as demands when the others believe they will be blamed or punished for not fulfilling the request.

It is human nature to want to help each other. We are designed to live in community and work as a team and help each other. So when a genuine request is made the listener will want to help with that request wherever possible and reasonable.

Putting It Together

So let's put these four steps together. Observation, feeling, need, request. Imagine the response you may get from, 'You don't support me in this process and it makes me sad, you don't care about me,' compared to, '[Observation] When I think about the fact you haven't come to the last three appointments [Feeling] I feel sad because I have a [Need] need to know we are united on this journey. [Request] Would it be possible to make sure the appointments are in your diary and nothing else gets added on those days?'

Which one do you think will lead to a more loving and unifying exchange?

Listening/Receiving Empathically.

When you understand the difference between thoughts and feelings, you can begin to see when others are communicating judgements and thoughts instead of owning their feelings. They are doing this out of all innocence.

Knowing this can enable the listener to not take things personally, to be able to respond compassionately. They can help seek to understand how the communicator is feeling, which builds empathy and mutual understanding.

Once the feeling has been identified then together they can then explore the need that isn't being met behind the feeling. You can begin to see how this can create a sense of unity when previously the exchange could have created discourse.

51

❖

Dialogue v discussion

The fertility journey can put a strain on the best of relationships. One of the gifts from our journey was that I learnt the importance of expressing and sharing emotions in a relationship. I wasn't aware how important it was for my wife to understand how I was feeling about things rather than what I thought about them. I also have a habit of being 'Mr Fix It' and all she craved was for me to understand how she felt, not fix it.

I want to share a communication strategy that I teach clients which can help couples feel more connected, united and ultimately more loved. Taking time to check in with each other and really understand how each other feel's about things is the glue that keeps us strong in difficult times. It's about holding a space for the other person to feel safe to express themselves without trying to change or judge their feelings. It is having a dialogue with each other rather than a discussion.

A discussion is a sharing of views, opinions and perspectives. A dialogue is seeking to understand the other person.

Common traits of a discussion

A discussion can often remain at a surface level for a number of reasons. Such as:

People can be thinking about how they are going to respond to what someone is saying more than deeply listening to what is being communicated.

A discussion can tend to be focussed on each person making their point, rather than seeking to deeply understand their partner. No-one likes to be wrong and we often end up protecting our corner more than understanding our partner.

Often there is not an acknowledgement or agreement to be totally focussed and real with each other, one party may be trying to get the discussion over as quickly as possible so they can get back to what they were doing or stop their partner 'going on'.

The benefits of dialoguing

Dialoguing, however, creates a safe and loving container for each person to share a deeper part of themselves and for the other person to understand and connect with them in that place.

Our partner is another person that lives in their own view of the world, which is probably very different to ours. Neither is right or wrong, just different. To truly understand someone you have to get out of your model of the world and in to theirs. This process can help you do that.

The dialoguing process

The Imago Dialogue is a unique three step process to create connection between two people. The depth of communication it fosters can have profound effects on a relationship.

In order to connect with someone deeply it can involve lowering our defence mechanisms. For me, it is coming out of my shell of thinking. I feel safe in there, no-one can hurt me emotionally, however it also prevents me from connecting more vulnerably and thus more deeply. Intimacy is sharing of oneself. So when I share more of myself to my wife I feel closer to her, more loved by her and more intimate with her.

In order to lower our defence mechanism we need to feel safe to do so. We don't feel safe to share our deepest selves if we fear we are going to be criticised, told we are wrong or shamed in any way. The Imago Dialogue process provides this safe container.

So the first rule is that here is no judgement, blame or criticism of your partner. Even if you feel really hurt by them this process gives you the structure to share how you feel without blame or judgement.

We do this by owning our feelings. No-one has the power to make you feel anything, you are experiencing your thinking about a situation not the situation itself. We focus on the feeling we want to share, not what/who we judge to be the cause of them. No-one is going to listen if they think they are about to be blamed or criticised.

We also do this by listening without judgement. It is easy for me to think my wife has misunderstood a situation and the feeling she is sharing is unnecessary. Listening without judgement is listening as if everything they are saying is absolutely true, because in their model of the world it *is* true for them. It is their 'reality' in this moment and that is what they want you to understand. Denying what they are saying is to deny their feelings in the moment.

Before you begin...

Agree when, and for how long, you are going to spend some time dialoguing and that it is the most important thing for you at that time.

Sit facing each other. Keep eye contact. Holding hands is a great way to remind yourself you are doing this to create a deeper understanding and connection.

Women are begging to be led my their man. I would suggest the man needs to lead this, to be responsible for making sure it happens, to lead his woman to the relationship she/you both inspire to have. The men are responsible for the 'container' of the relationship. Creating a space for the woman to be free to be the feminine energy they are.

The three steps.

1. Mirroring

One person shares his/her feelings or experiences to the other, owning the feeling by saying "I feel …" A useful phrase to use might be 'When I think about X, I feel…' It is sharing a feeling, not a thought, judgement or criticism and owning it. We can be lazy with our language and use the words 'I feel' but what tends to follow is a thought or judgement rather than a feeling. Make sure it is a feeling not a judgement. Make sure you are not blaming something/someone for the feeling. 'When I think about X, I feel' not 'When you said X it made me feel'.

The listener's job is to listen with the intent to understand, not to respond.

In response the listener plays back the words, either word for word or paraphrasing, to demonstrate they have heard. They could start by saying 'Let me see if I have got you. You said…'

The listener could then ask 'Is there more?' This helps the sharer explore if there is anything else they want share on the subject. Give them space to consider whether there is more. This demonstrates to your partner you are open to what they have to say, whatever it is. If they share more, again demonstrate you have heard by playing back what they have said to give them an opportunity to check you have got it all.

Some mirroring phrases:

'Let me see if I've got it…', 'I heard you say…', 'Did I get that?', 'Is there more?'

2. Validation

This step is to acknowledge their experience verbally so they hear it. Validation is verbally acknowledging their experience as being valid, i.e. not telling them it is necessary or they are silly for feeling that way or trying to correct them in any way.

You don't have to agree with them to validate their experience. Remember you are getting in to their model of the world and seeing things from their perspective/mindset in that moment and acknowledging the reality of it for them. If something doesn't make sense you can ask for clarity on what doesn't make sense but without judgement or whether it is right or wrong.

When your validate your partner you can often see a shift in their energy and their way of being as they feel accepted.

Some validation phrases:

'That makes sense to be because...', 'I can understand that given that...', 'I can see how you would see it that way because...'

3. Empathy

So far the listener has demonstrated they have heard their partner without judgement. The next step is in some ways the crown jewels. It is going deeper from 'hearing' someone to 'understanding' them. More importantly it is *demonstrating* that you understand. You cannot say 'I understand how you feel', only the sharer can say 'you understand' when you have demonstrated you understand.

We can all have a different experience of what we mean when we use a word. Once my wife and I both said we felt angry about a situation. When we unpacked it she was livid and I was annoyed. We both had a very different experience even though we had used the same word.

Empathy is demonstrating you understand their *experience*

behind their words. Don't listen to what they are saying, feel in to the energy of what they mean behind the words.

The best place to start is to play-back how you think they are feeling in your own words. 'I imagine you are feeling scared right now, is that right?' Find out how strong the feeling is, perhaps on a scale of 1 to 10. Perhaps think of a time you felt the same feeling in your life. 'Is it like the time I was scared I was going to lose my job?' This gives your partner an opportunity to refine your understanding of their experience. They may say yes, that's just it, but 100 times stronger. Or they may say 'no it's not like that, it's like the time we got lost in the dark on the walk in the hills'.

The questioning and exploring helps refine your understanding of their experience behind the words, which demonstrates to them that you really understand how they feel.

At the end you can check to see if there is anything else you could have acknowledged but didn't.

Some empathy phrases:

'I imagine you might be feeling… Is that right?', 'Is like [metaphor]', 'Is it like the time I…'

How to use it

You can do this for a particular issue you are facing in your life at that time or just as a way of checking in with each other and connecting at a deeper level.

You can do it both ways and switch roles or do it one way.

Have fun connecting and feeling more united. I know it may not feel like it but there can be some amazing gifts for you on this rollercoaster and I hope that a deeper connection between you and your partner is one of them.

52

Love languages

Have you ever been in a situation where someone just doesn't get what you are saying and you can't see why? We are all unique and experience the world in through our thoughts, beliefs and understanding. We all have our own models of the world. For our communication to be successful we need to ensure we are communicating in a way that the recipient understands. In a way which fits with their model of the world, which can be quite different to ours. The same is true when it comes to love. So a pertinent question might be, "are you communicating love to your partner/loved ones in a way they understand it?"

After more than 20 years of experience, relationship counsellor Gary Chapman identified five typical ways in which we tend to give and receive love. These are outlined in his book *The Five Love Languages*. Unconsciously we each have a preference as to the ways in which we receive love. The thing is, we tend to express love to others in the same way that we prefer to receive it but that may not be the same way our partner prefers to receive it! Our 'love languages' may be as different as English and Chinese and no matter how hard we try to express love in English, if our partner only understands Chinese, our act of love will be lost in the translation and, more likely than not, leave us feeling unloved and not appreciated.

Understanding each other's 'love language' enables you to show love in ways each other appreciate and the results can transform a relationship.

Another good thing about this is that it only takes one person in the relationship to understand the language of their partner to bring more love into the relationship. If your partner is feeling more loved they are more likely to reciprocate and be more loving back.

We all like to receive love in a whole manner of ways but we tend to have a primary preference, like being right or left handed. One way that stands out as making the biggest impact on us when receiving love.

OK, so what are the love languages? Like with spoken language there are various 'dialects' within each love language so it's important to understand what dialect your partner has in their primary love language.

1. Words of Affirmation.

The love language of Words of Affirmation has dialects within it such as compliments, encouragement, affirmation and kindness.

Compliments can be anything from simple compliments such as telling them that you think they look nice or thanking them for something. Words of encouragement or affirmations can be powerful as we all have untapped potential or areas where we feel insecure which may be transformed by our partner's words. It might be kind words or tone of voice. How often do we communicate by the tone of our voice rather than with our actual words, using a harsh tone when we're angry or frustrated, rather than expressing our feelings in a gentler tone?

Another dialect is not the giving words of affirmation but the absence of criticism. This is true for me. Compliments by-pass me quickly whereas criticism cuts deep and stays with me. This also means if I am not careful I can habitually be slow at giving my wife compliments (but never criticise her).

2. Quality Time.

Quality Time has dialects such as undivided attention, shared activities, listening and sharing.

Undivided attention means focussing on each other without any distractions. It may not be staring into each other eyes, it could be sharing an activity together that has a sense of cooperation or camaraderie. When a parent rolls a ball to a toddler it is not about the activity itself, but the connection that is created between them.

My wife and I sometimes find that holding hands when we are talking is a means of demonstrating that we are giving each other our undivided attention – something important to my wife as this is her primary love language!

It may not just be talking, it might well be quality activities; doing something with your partner that you know they will enjoy wholeheartedly, even if you do not particularly like the activity. For example, perhaps you partner likes going to the ballet but you prefer action films! You could suggest going to the ballet together. It can become a quality time activity if one party wants to do it and the other party is willing to join in order to express love by being with each other.

Quality time also involves quality conversation. This requires learning to listen as well as learning to talk. Listening for what is really being communicated rather than what we think is being communicated (or jumping in with solutions as men like to do). It also requires learning to share how we feel not just what we think. That leads to quality conversation and a connection.

3. Gifts.

Gary Chapman studied anthropology visiting and studying a huge number of groups all over the world. In every culture, he found that gift-giving was part of their love/marriage ceremony (e.g. rings). Giving and receiving gifts can be a means of expressing love and for some people, it is their primary love language.

When someone gives a gift they are generally thinking of the recipient when they obtain it. You can look at a gift and it can remind you of the person who gave it to you and the fact that they remembered or thought of you enough to give a gift.

Again there are a number of dialects in the language of gifts such as the expensive gifts, home-made tokens of love or gifts of your time. Gifts can be extravagant or simple, they can be bought, made or found; from huge and expensive displays of affection to the single daisy we picked on the way home because we were thinking of our partner.

A friend of ours was snorkelling on his honeymoon and came out of the water minus his wedding ring. His new bride made him go back in and would not let him out until he found it. He quickly learned that gifts was her primary love language (and thankfully he found the ring!).

4. Acts of Service.

The dialects within acts of service are doing what is important to your partner. This is doing something you know your partner would like you to do – not what you think is important or what you want to do!

I do lots of things around the house like maintaining the car and computer but these things can often fail to register with my wife. However, if I clean the bathroom it gets noticed!

This can often challenge our stereotypical roles for men and women which may come from the assumed roles our parents played. The trick is knowing what is important for your partner, not just what to do but how to do it. My taking the rubbish out doesn't have the same impact for my wife as cleaning the bathroom. For my wife I know she has a far greater attention to detail than myself so when I do something for her I know I need to take more care and ensure I am doing it as if she would – without my short-cuts! So cleaning the bathroom to her standards, not mine!

5. Physical Touch.

Touch is a powerful way of communicating emotional love. What do we often do in a time of crisis to demonstrate love? We hug someone. Touch can communicate love or hate. A caress can be life-enhancing and tender, a push or shove can be devastating.

Men often think this is their primary love language because of their love of sex. One question I ask is would you want sex with your partner if they had been criticising you all day? Or if they had ignored you all day? If the answer is no then perhaps Physical Touch is not your primary love language.

The dialects within physical touch can be explicit touch such as massage where you are focussed on the act of touch, or it could be implicit such as a glancing touch as you brush past your partner or reach for something.

Understanding Your Primary Love Language.

Just reading the explanations above may give you an indication of what you and your partner's primary love languages might be. In addition, here are some questions that may help you to identify your primary love language:

- What does your partner do that hurts you most deeply?

- What have you most often requested from your partner?
- In what ways do you regularly express love to your partner?

If you find it difficult to identify your primary love language it could be that you have felt loved for some time through a variety of love languages making it difficult to identify which is the key one for you. Or that you haven't felt loved for some time and you cannot remember which one makes the difference to you. If this is the case try asking yourself:

- What did you like about your partner when you fell in love with them?
- What would your ideal partner be like?

Communicating love to your partner in their preferred love language can transform a relationship as they will feel emotionally loved and wanted. They will automatically respond and reflect that love back to you. Give it a go. See if you can identify your partner's primary love language. Do something to express your love to them in that way every day for two weeks. Watch the transformation unfold.

Part 6

Putting it together

53

❖

Answering the dreaded question

I initially wrote 'What to do if asked if you're going to have children' as the chapter title. I then changed it to what to do when someone asks because I'm pretty sure it is inevitable that someone will ask at some point. Particularly if you are of the age when many of your peers are having children. The inevitability of it can make some situations uncomfortable. The idea of being the odd one out and people wondering why.

Being asked this question can lead to one feeling awkward, confused as to what to say and bring up the pain and despair of the journey all over again.

So how can we be comfortable with being asked this question? On our journey we found a way of approaching this that took away the fear of being asked and have more peace of mind with how we responded and not having to think on our feet when our mind has gone to mush as it can do when overwhelmed with emotion (that's because we can't think and feel at the same time!).

Fearing the Dreaded Question

There may be times you are dreading the question being asked. You perhaps are wondering whether people are asking the question in their own minds and when they are actually going to ask you for real.

This fear of being asked is based on an expectation of how you may find that future experience. How you expect to feel if you are asked. It may be based on past experiences but it's still an imaginary image/movie in your head of how you expect it may go and how you may feel at being asked. It is future thinking taking you away from being present and grounded.

There's a couple of things I want to explore about these future scenarios playing over in our heads.

Firstly, they are fantasy. Remember it's the future and the future doesn't exist. It only exists in our thinking. Yes, what you are imagining may be totally realistic and based on past experience but nothing can predict the future, not even your thinking. We often think of fantasy as un-realistic things, such as pigs flying! However, any thought that is not in the present moment is pure fantasy as it doesn't exist. It is made up.

Another thing to remember is that the 'us' in that imagined future in our head is not the fully resourced us. As a species, human beings are designed to be in the moment, in reality, not our la-la land future in our head. We have an amazing range of resources to enable us to deal with reality, whatever life throws up at us when we are in it. We have innate well-being, emotional resilience, wisdom, creativity, insight, clarity, perspective etc. etc. when we are in reality. When we are in our imagined future in our heads these are not present. So no wonder it feels scary or we think we wouldn't be able to cope with that imagined scenario. This is why rehearsing future scenarios in our head is not always useful.

This future thinking creates an expectation which puts us on edge and into our heads even before we've got to the reality of being asked. This prevents us from being present and grounded even before we have been asked.

Having Peace of Mind

Being asked whether we are going to have children and the many unhelpful things our friends and family tend to say can trigger an emotional response within you. Well, it can appear to work that way. It's not actually the question or what has been said that is making you feel anything. If we think it is the question that makes us feel upset then no wonder we want to avoid being asked and find it difficult to answer.

What if you could remember that 100% of our human experience comes from Thought in the moment? Everything we experience as a human being comes from Thought. Thought is the creator of our experience, but then says it didn't do it! It leads us to believe it was the circumstances, what someone had just said, that created our experience. Nothing has the power to make us feel anything. We live in the experience of our thinking 100% of the time. It doesn't work any other way.

So the first thing is to remember where you experience is coming from. It's not coming from what you can see, the circumstances in front of you, in life. It's coming from the stories you are telling yourself in that moment about those circumstances.

It's nothing to do with what has been asked, or who has asked it, it's what you are telling yourself.

If you find yourself being emotional at being asked, you've taken yourself on a journey, probably into the future and imagining the future without children, reliving your fear of not getting pregnant. You are no longer present, in reality, where your innate well-being and resourcefulness exist.

Agree on a Strategy

We found it really helpful to agree what we would say to people when asked. We personally found being honest was the best way to avoid further embarrassment and questions. We agreed that if someone were to ask if we are going to have children we would say 'we would love to be we are not sure we are able to' without giving any further details or indicating who the 'difficulties' may lie with.

In our experience, the person asking the question found the situation and response more awkward than we did. It didn't lead to in-depth questions or interrogations, and it enabled us to accept the reality of the situation and know we can handle it rather than avoiding the reality which in fact can make it worse.

A Native American approach to painful situations is to tell as many people as possible your story and find gradually the emotion diminishes each time you share it. It doesn't change the reality of the situation but can take out any intense emotion tied up in it.

So I recommend you agree with your partner what you will both say when asked about having children. This also enables you to know that both of you are singing from the same song-sheet, both using a script you are happy with.

You may find with this understanding of what is happening psychologically and a prepared approach you're not so scared of people asking the question and when they do you're more at peace as you respond.

54

❖

They're everywhere!

Why is it that when you choose what car you are going to buy you suddenly see more of them on the road? When I was training as a hypnotherapist our trainer used to do a group hypnosis session at the end of the day to help cement the learning from that day. He used to have some fun by adding that we would be surprised at how many Minis we saw on our journey home. This always surprised me at how it worked! I used to get the tube home but even in my short walk to the station at either end, I was aware of Minis everywhere in the traffic! This is called priming. We are more likely to see what our mind has been primed to see. It's subconsciously looking for them or noticing them more than any other car.

There's a famous experiment you can find on YouTube where there are two small teams passing a basketball between them, interweaving between themselves as they do. One team is in white, the other in black. You are asked to count how many times the white team pass the ball. What most people don't notice is the black gorilla that walks through the scene, does a little dance and then moves on! They have been primed to notice only the white people and everything else gets tuned out of their awareness.

There is a phrase, 'the more you focus on, the more you get'. My mind was primed to see Minis. It was focussing on Minis so it could make the match and identify them when it saw one. Your mind is pretty much constantly on your infertility journey and how much you want a baby. So guess what, what do you see more of? Pregnant women and babies. Pretty tough eh?

For me, seeing fathers with their young children was really tough for me. It was a trigger for Outside-In Thought leading to feeling despair, anger and sadness.

So, what can you do about it? Well, the more you see through the illusion of Outside-In Thought, that really believes your psychological well-being and happiness is dependant on having a baby, the less your mind is thinking about it and thus you are not so primed to see them. The more we know what is creating our experience, Thought, the less we get tricked by the illusion and the greater clarity and perspective we have moment to moment that sees a wider range of opportunities in our life and in any given moment. It's not fixated on having a baby.

Secondly, be aware in what way are you making someone else's pregnancy about you? This is what Outside-In Thought does. It makes everything about us when it actually isn't. The emotional response comes from the story you are telling yourself that makes someone else being pregnant about you. Perhaps 'it's never going to happen to me'. Notice the situation is not about you and also how do you know these stories are true? Really true? You will probably find they are all future stories and remember nothing can predict the future.

If you have frequently had a negative reaction to seeing someone pregnant it becomes what's called an anchor. An anchor is a link between a situation and an emotional response. The missing link between them is Thought but it happens so quickly it's an immediate trigger of response from the situation or even memory. For example, often a smell may take you back to memories of childhood. That's an anchor, a link between the memory and a smell.

You can actively create positive anchors. For example, if you find public speaking difficult and it is a necessary part of your job you can spend time imagining speaking and seeing it going really well. You can imagine feeling great whilst doing it and associate this feeling and experience with either a physical sensation, e.g. A gentle squeeze of a knuckle or a particular smell, e.g. an essential oil or favourite perfume. The more you spend time associating that experience with the squeeze or smell the stronger it gets. So when you come to speak you can either breathe in your smell or a give a subtle squeeze of your knuckle and the nerves are replaced with that confidence you felt when you imagined that great talk creating the anchor.

Remember, your mind cannot tell the difference between imagination and reality so the emotions you feel when you imagine speaking with confidence are the real thing, your mind becomes familiar with it and can recall it more easily when you need it. I had a client who used her favourite perfume and before we went to speak would take a big breath of it in (having put some on just beforehand) as she walked up to speak. It transformed her state into one of confidence.

You could do this with seeing pregnant women. Imagine what you would want to feel. Perhaps hopeful or confident that it is going to be you one day. This sounds strange but imagine your head on the other person's body, notice how that feels, then make it your head and your (pregnant) body. Turn them into a pregnant you and experience how it feels. Use the situation to remind your unconscious mind what you want instead of the Outside-In stories that usually fill your mind.

This is a fabulous way to turn that negative experience into something more positive for you, and your fertility. As you practice that you may be surprised how different you feel next time you see one out and about. It helps your thinking switch from 'it's never going to happen for me' or 'it's not fair', which are all victim states, to 'this is what I am heading towards, I'm not there yet but we are on the journey', which is moving from a victim state to creator state.

55

❖

How to survive another BFN

We've all been in the depths on this roller-coaster. Your period coming on can trigger a dive down into a dip. Perhaps you can anticipate it, reading the signals in your body. The fear and dread building up. The heartbreak when it does. Imagining that it's never going to happen for you, that you don't have the strength to carry on but can't imagine giving up.

There is no right or wrong way of dealing with another negative test result (Big Fat Negative) as we are all unique and experience things in different ways but I want to share with you some things that may or may not be coming up for you.

Understanding what you are feeling

The text I got from my wife had no meaning until I gave it meaning. The competitor moving in across the street means nothing until I give it meaning. The downturn in the housing market means nothing until I create a meaning for it, and so, therefore, all these feelings that prevent me from having peace of mind and hope for the future have been caused by my thoughts, not by events or circumstances.

Events cannot cause feelings, they just don't have that power. It's not how our mind works. The biological computer that is our mind processes thoughts. That's it. Thoughts. We live in the experience of our thinking, nothing else. Our feeling doesn't know anything about our circumstances and they definitely don't know anything about the future because the future doesn't exist, except in our thinking.

It definitely feels like it is coming from the circumstances and you are feeling your situation, but that is the illusion of thought and feelings. In the same way it "feels like" the earth is flat and it "feels like" the sun goes away at night. We misinterpret a lot until we understand how things really work. Until we understand we are only ever feeling our thinking we shall be chasing our tail of thinking and getting more and more caught up in the rollercoaster of emotions.

Pain passes because thinking moves on

The thing about feelings is that because they are created by our thoughts and by the nature of thoughts they come and go feelings cannot stay forever, although it can feel like they do. We look at a situation through a set of thinking, a state of mind. It is like looking at a situation through a long cardboard tube (e.g. wrapping paper tube). We see a perspective. Imagine there is a vertical stack of tubes one on top of the other. We may be looking at the situation through the lowest tube, the lowest level of consciousness. We think that is 'reality' unaware that we have the capability of seeing the situation (and thus experiencing it) through any other level of consciousness (thinking) at any given moment. This is why sometimes things feel better than others. Our circumstances haven't changed but the meaning we give them (our thinking) has.

Thinking comes and it goes by its nature. You couldn't hold on to a feeling (even anger at your partner!) forever even if you wanted to. They say time heals all wounds. That is not actually correct. Time doesn't heal anything because we are only ever feeling our thinking – it is the changes in our thinking over time that changes our experience.

It's not your fault

Often after an IVF failure clients can tend to blame themselves for it not working. They think that perhaps if they had looked after themselves more or taken more supplements or this/that/the other things may be different. Our brain likes reasons for things. By nature, it is a pattern hunter which is why it is possible to read sentenecs wtih radnom lettres in teh worng odrer.

The truth is fertility is an art as well as a science. If it were a pure science you wouldn't be reading this as the scientists would have it cracked 100% by now. Sometimes on paper a couple have absolutely no reason why things shouldn't work and they don't. Conversely, you have couples that on paper shouldn't have a hope in hell of getting pregnant and they do.

The doctors often learn something about your body on each cycle so may have some recommendations for future treatment, other than that stop looking for reasons, it doesn't serve you as you tend to lose perspective when you go down that route. You end up chasing your thinking tail.

Predicting the future

Our thinking has a habit of telling us what something means for our future. When your period starts it is easy to get caught into the story of what that means for your future, about whether you will ever have children, will you ever find true happiness and fulfilment?

The thing is, nothing can predict the future not even your thinking. You have no idea what is going to happen in the next five minutes let alone next month or next year. Our thinking plays an imaginary movie of the future in our mind that so plausible and believable we forget it's a movie, that it's made up. Any thought that is not in the present moment is pure fantasy. We often think of fantasy as unrealistic things like people flying. However, any thought that is not in the present moment is pure fantasy.

Come back to the here and now, that's where you'll find peace of mind, perspective and clarity about what is next for you.

Innate well-being

There is a space below your thinking that is behind your pain and anguish. That space is your soul that knows you are OK whatever happens. That's your innate well-being. It's what you access when you have a quiet mind, present to the moment and not caught in the stories in your head about what it means for your future happiness that your period has started.

That innate well-being is there whether we recognise it in the moment or not. Sometimes we go Outside-In, that's OK, it's called being human. But know when you feel despair and pain it will pass. It's Thought in this moment and it will pass. It's not you or the situation, I know it really feels like it is. Allow yourself to feel the pain, you don't need to be scared of it or get caught up in it. Don't resent it or wish it wasn't there. Allow it knowing it's stories you are telling yourself in this moment and they will pass. Self-compassion is the order of the day.

I shared this metaphor for how our innate well-being is there whether we know it or not in even in the depths of despair in chapter 27. I want you to read it again.

Imagine that you are riding on a giant barge, floating gently down a beautiful river. In the very centre of the barge is a giant roller coaster, and your seat for the journey is in the front car. As the river carries the barge downstream, the roller coaster goes up and down, pausing every now and again before climbing its way to the next peak or plunging its way down into the valleys. At times it spins wildly, completely disorienting you, at other times you find yourself resting in the pause before the next ride.

Now imagine that your whole life you had ridden the coaster with your eyes closed, believing that the roller coaster was the world and the river only a myth. What would happen the first time you opened your eyes and kept them open for every moment of the ride?

At first, you might be a bit disoriented and even frightened as you watched yourself and others go up and down and round and around at occasionally dizzying speeds. The first time you crested the heights of the coaster and saw the river clearly in all its glory, you would be so taken by the view that you would never want it to end. And when your revelation was followed by a plunge to the bottom of your world it might seem like all was lost.

But over time, you would begin to relax into the ride, spending less and less time trying to manage the ups and downs and more and more time enjoying the views along the way. You'd take comfort in the fact that no matter what was going on with the roller coaster, the river was always effortlessly supporting the barge along its journey. And you might even begin to enjoy pondering the mysteries of where the river came from, how you came to be on it, and where it might be taking you...

Whatever happens you are going to be OK. Let go of those future-thinking stories based on fear. Come back to the here and now. You have everything you need to be OK in this moment. Breathe back into this moment. Tomorrow will take care of itself.

56

❖

How to survive IVF

The fertility journey is often referred to as an emotional rollercoaster. Undergoing fertility treatment such as IVF is one hell of a ride! It can feel like many years of the fertility journey are condensed into a month. So how do you survive this? How can you move from survival to feel like your body is thriving?

Whatever happens, you'll be OK

The first thing is to let go of the outcome. It's to know whatever happens you will be OK. There's nothing wrong with wanting to have a baby. The more we hold the outcome lightly in one hand and in the other hand know we are OK whatever happens, the creative energy between the two moves us forward towards success with greater ease and well-being. Whatever it is in life we want to achieve, whether it's IVF success or career success it is possible with greater ease and well-being when we know that there is nothing we need to be OK psychologically. We came into the world as a soul that is complete and perfect. It's out contaminated Outside-In Thought that we pick up over the years that thinks our OKness is in some way dependant on something in this physical world. Either we need to be different or our circumstances need to be different. This is an illusion. If we chase the thing we think we need it doesn't scratch the itch, there will always be something else. Needing something is fuelled by a fear of not getting it and thus not being OK. Desiring it is knowing we are OK whatever happens. If you don't know this re-read the book and see what else you take from it that helps you see through the illusion of Outside-In Thought and collect more deeply to your innate well-being.

Use the power of visualisation

For IVF success you need three things:

1. A good quality embryo.
2. A healthy environment for the embryo to be placed in.
3. A healthy interaction between the embryo and your uterus.

Given our unconscious mind controls all our bodily functions and we have access to it you have the ability to give it a helping hand to create the biological circumstances to maximise success. Throughout each stage of the treatment imagine your body doing exactly what you wanted to do at that stage.

Stimulation

For example, during stimulation imagine your body responding to, and working in harmony with, the medication. Visualise the medication doing what it needs to do in a healthy balanced way for you and your body. Use whatever images or metaphors come to mind and that represent what you want to happen within you.

Egg collection

As you approach egg collection imagine your body harvesting a large number of good quality eggs in whichever way your imagination sees that. One client imagined the good quality eggs within her being red and the poor quality ones being blue. She imagined a sea of dots to represent her eggs within her and imagined more and more being red than blue. When she did this she harvested a much higher number of good quality eggs on her next IVF than the previous one. Was that purely down to this visualisation? Who knows, but she believes it was a significant factor and it helped her feel like she could be doing something useful in the process instead of just worrying about it.

Embryo Transfer

As you approach embryo transfer, imagine your body creating the safest most welcoming place for the embryo. Remember how the uterus wall welcomes the embryo and wraps the lining around it, it's not purely down to the embryo 'embedding' itself in. Your body is welcoming and embracing it. How would you imagine that happening within you? What else could you imagine that represents your body welcoming your embryo(s)?

Be as relaxed as possible during the embryo transfer. Remember the study from chapter 36 that showed being relaxed during embryo transfer can significantly increase the success rate. Listen to something on your phone/mp3 player. Don't be rushed before or afterwards. Imagine your body welcoming the embryo.

The 2 Week Wait deserves a chapter of its own!

Keep talking

It's an emotional rollercoaster and can be a very stressful experience. Ensure you and your partner are talking beyond surface level conversation. Use the dialogue process in chapter 51 to ensure you stay connected, united and feeling fully supported. Remember at times of stress the typical male and female reactions to stress can mean we feel more disconnected and frustrated with each other. Don't take things personally. Anything said in a low state of mind can be ignored, it's not coming from their true self. Take conscious action to stay connected.

You are not alone

Often women and couples go through IVF and they consciously decide not to tell people. This can be because they know others don't really understand what it's like on this journey and they decide they are probably better off without their well-meaning but misguided comments. It can also be to take the pressure off themselves so people are not asking how it is going and there is less pressure on the outcome. Whatever the motivation, it can often be a lonely journey. I encourage you to find support somewhere beyond your partner. At least one other woman you can talk to and be real with. This may be someone physical or it could be supported via an online support forum such as Fertility Friends. In the UK there is also support from Fertility Network UK which has an online forum and fertility nurse helpline. In the US there is the support of the fertility charity, Resolve.

Whatever happens, you are going to be OK.

57

❖

How to thrive in the 2WW

I originally called this chapter how to survive the two-week wait as that is what most people want to know. There is an expectation (perhaps based on past experience) that it is going to be a stressful ordeal. Absolutely, the two-week wait can be an incredibly stressful and lonely experience.

If you've had fertility treatment such as IVF, the clinic has been guiding you through the process and caring for you along the way. Suddenly you get to the point at which they have done all they can. It can feel like it's now down to you. No pressure then! You can suddenly feel alone and not sure what to do. You feel the pressure is on you and your body to perform.

If you are trying naturally it is the constant and regular nervousness of whether this is the month that your dreams come true, and the dread of it not being the case. The constant fear of your period coming on and being over-sensitive to signals in your body. Thinking you cannot take another month of the emotional rollercoaster and not being pregnant.

However, it doesn't have to be that way.

Even the term 'two-week wait' implies it is a wait. Waiting for something you don't yet have.

If you have IVF, the truth is you are pregnant from the moment of embryo transfer. Too many people forget that and are so focussed on the upcoming test result they forget the reality of where they are in this moment. I once had a conversation with a lady who had IVF in the pioneering times of the early 1980s. Back then success rates were far lower and they monitored you more closely after embryo transfer. She said it was like entering a lottery. She knew the odds were low. When she was told she was pregnant, at a very early stage and not to get her hopes up, she told everyone! She thought she may never have another opportunity to say the words 'I'm pregnant'. She went on to have twins! I suspect her embracing the moment may have had a part in that. She was not full of fear, her body could relax and a relaxed uterus is key to IVF success.

If you are trying naturally your body doesn't go on hold until you take a pregnancy test. If you freeze in fear, your body will freeze as well.

Waiting is all about focussing on a future event. During your journey up to this point, it's all been about focussing on an outcome, something you've been hoping for for a long time – in the future. You may feel like your life has been on hold, focussing so much on Project Baby. Perhaps you have given up work to focus on your lifestyle and reduce stress. Your fertility and treatment have been the main focus of your life and the rest of life can seem to shrink or disappear.

This pressure and waiting can be even more heightened and exaggerated during the two-week wait. Like holding a breath for two weeks waiting to know whether you have succeeded and are going to be OK.

Stress and anxiety all come from future thinking. And waiting is all about future thinking. When we recognise where we are, in this moment, and let go of future thinking we let go of stress and anxiety. We are human 'beings'. Designed to 'be' in the now. The only moment that exists in time is the present moment.

It's about reframing the whole experience and expectation of the two-week wait. The two-week wait is not a wait. It is a period of time to allow your body to thrive in what it is actively doing in that moment. It is a period of time to allow your body to embrace your embryo(s) and pregnancy.

Your thinking wants you to be pregnant so much, it is so scared you may not get it, perhaps it is trying to prevent you from being disappointed, bracing yourself in case it is bad news. All that is well intended, however, it is all future thinking which creates stress and tension in your mind and body and not a place for you and your embryo(s) to thrive.

Turn the Two Week Wait into a Two Week Thrive by trusting where you are is perfect for you. Imagine your body doing what it needs to do in each moment. At this moment right now, not what may or may not be when you take the test. Tomorrow can take care of itself, being there today with your body, as that is where it is! Your future thinking disconnects you from your body, come back and breathe life into your body and connect with it in this moment.

Visualise your body doing what you want to do in each moment. Be with your body in this moment. Connect with it. Put your hand on your womb and breathe into that space. What do you want it to know? If it could tell you something what would it want to tell you?

Take each day as it comes. Be with your body, it lives in the present moment. Be aware your mind may time travel but reality and your body are in the here and now. Love and connect with it.

To help you do this I suggest a daily reflection period where each day you do three things.

1. Write down three things you are grateful for. Gratitude is a powerful thing and it opens you up to recognise what you have in

your life instead of focussing on what you haven't got. It connects you to the energy of receiving and not being stuck in the energy of needing. These three things could be something as small as seeing something in nature. They don't need to be grand things but things or moments you are thankful for. The gifts in our day or life we often take for granted.

2. Spend a few minutes connecting with your body. Put your hand on your womb and breathe into that space. Imagine what's happening in there and what you want to happen. If your body or womb could say something to you in this moment what might it be? Write it down.

3. Think about what you are going to do that day or in the next 24hrs for you. As a gesture of love for yourself. Write that down by using this structure. Start with the words 'I promise you…[what you will do]…because I said I would.' Make that a promise to yourself.

Use this daily reflection to ground yourself to the here and now. You may find dipping into this book, picking a chapter at random or one that speaks to you as a way of reminding yourself that the fear and distress are Thought in this moment. They don't know anything about the future. Come back to the here and now. It's there you'll know whatever happens you are going to be OK.

58

❖

Secondary Infertility

I wanted to write a quick note about secondary infertility. The first thing is that, like any infertility, most friends and family do not understand the considerable stress and distress that can be experienced. I would say this is even more so when it comes to secondary infertility. People think that as you have a child/ children already it means that it is not as painful and difficult as when experiencing infertility with no children. However this is not always the case. It can be just as painful. Don't let other people's expectations of what they think you are experiencing make you feel bad or wrong for feeling what you are feeling. Feelings are spontaneous and never good, bad, right or wrong.

In my experience a high percentage of secondary infertility are the result of trauma or distress associated with the birth (or time soon after) of the first child or miscarriage. If this is the case your unconscious mind may be trying to protect you from a similar experience. It unconsciously equates getting pregnant to trauma or distress. Of course we know consciously this is not universally the case however the unconscious mind is there to protect you and sometimes is over-protective and is scared the same thing may happen again.

If you did experienced distress during a previous birth or in the early days of motherhood (e.g. postnatal depression) I encourage you to seek a therapist or counsellor to help you let go

of that trauma. You may be able to rationalise it but your unconscious mind and body may be holding on to the distress and
fear unnecessarily. If you have strong emotions when you think
about the previous birth it probably means there is some letting
go that could take place. I encourage you to seek a Cognitive
Hypnotherapist (www.qchpa.com) who can help you clear any
underlying fear.

59

❖

My Wish For You

I hope that you've found the book helpful and my wish for you is that it begins a new chapter in your journey and your life. That you can truly know you are OK whatever happens, on the journey and in life and this opens up a feeling of peace from which the magic can happen.

I've said it before but I wouldn't wish a 10 year fertility journey on anyone, but I hope you've got a glimpse of what I learned about myself and life that you can begin to see in your own life, and perhaps see the gifts for you on your journey that will stay with you forever and help you be the parent you would love to be.

To download some free resources to help you further on your journey and to get some inspiration straight to your inbox, sign up on my website www.thefertilemind.net. It would be lovely to stay in touch and support you further on your journey to parenthood. You can find some hypnosis programmes to download and can contact me directly via the website.

I wish you every success on your fertility journey and enjoy connecting to the wonder of your true self.

With love
Russell x

Recommend Reading

If you would like some recommended reading to take some of the ideas and principles from this book further, here is a list of books I recommend.

Mindset
How To Master Anxiety by Joe Griffin and Ivan Tyrrell
Clarity by Jamie Smart
The Inside Out Revolution by Michael Neill
Somebody Should Have Told Us by Jack Pransky
The Enlightened Gardner by Sydney Banks
Stop Thinking Start Living by Richard Carlson
Daring Greatly by Brené Brown,

Mind-Body Link
Biology of Belief by Bruce Lipton
It's the Thought That Counts by Dr David Hamilton
How Your Mind Can Heal Your Body by Dr David Hamilton

Relationships
The Relationship Handbook by George Pransky
The Way Of The Superior Man by David Deida
The Five Love Languages by Gary Chapman
Non Violent Communication by Marshall Rosenberg

About Russell

Russell Davis is a Coach and Cognitive Hypnotherapist, writer and speaker and helps people remove psychological blocks to getting pregnant. Russell's personal experience echoes his belief that too many couples go through fertility treatment unnecessarily and that the success rate of treatment is unnecessarily low. Whether natural or assisted conception, Russell has helped hundreds of couples all over the world move from despair to hope to success.

Russell founded The Fertile Mind fertility mind-body programs and coaching based on his and his wife's 10-year double infertility journey which resulted in the natural conception of their son. Russell's primary focus is to help people to have less on their minds and connect to their true sense of self and the amazing resources and innate well-being with them.

Russell lives in the UK and when he's not working with clients or writing he loves getting out into nature barefoot running, kayaking and working on cars.

Find out more about Russell and his work at www.thefertilemind.net.

23546046R00142

Printed in Great Britain
by Amazon